the
Quick & Clean
Diet

Lose the Weight, Feel Great, and Stay Lean for Life

Dari Alexander
Foreword by Dr. Mehmet Oz

Guilford, Connecticut

An imprint of Globe Pequot Press

To buy books in quantity for corporate use
or incentives, call **(800) 962-0973**
or e-mail **premiums@GlobePequot.com.**

Text design: Sheryl Kober
Layout: Casey Shain
Project editor: Ellen Urban
Nutrition consultant: Karen Konopelski Hensley MS, RD, CSSD

Library of Congress Cataloging-in-Publication Data is available on file.

ISBN 978-0-7627-8172-0

Printed in the United States of America

10 9 8 7 6 5 4 3 2 1

To my incredibly patient and loving husband, Will,
and to my adorable babies, Dex and Scarlett Rose.
I only began to live when you all came into my life.

Contents

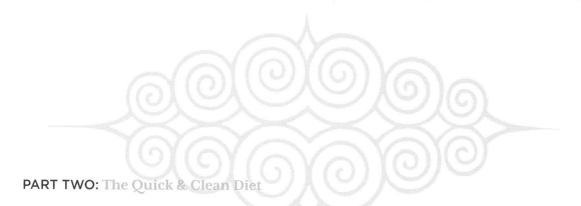

Foreword

Much of my life has been spent wrestling with the hearts of patients damaged by years of lifestyle missteps. Most of the hypertension, diabetes, and high cholesterol that rusts the insides of our bodies is caused by a single, clever culprit—obesity. I also see the struggles many have in achieving their desired weight while juggling commitments to work and family. All too often people are drawn to extreme diet plans that lead to frustration and a yo-yo pattern of weight loss and gain that is devastating to health. Part pep talk, part nutrition, *The Quick & Clean Diet* is a gentle yet effective approach to sustained weight loss that will guide you through the emotional process of meeting your weight loss goal. Dari Alexander's voice resonates for me because she understands firsthand the practical trade-offs required for a sustainable lifestyle change. She understands that dieting is not a wind sprint, but rather a marathon.

I first met Dari Alexander on-air, as she interviewed me for a news story for her job in broadcast television. She is fit, smart, and naturally curious, with a passion for health. Her children reflect her enthusiastic quest for wellness, and their natural proclivity to eat well reflects Dari's ability to create a home where eating the right food is easy to do. We have since become friends, and I admire her abilities as a journalist and her passion for her family. Dari is a working mom who knows what it's like to feel the pressure to lose weight and to fail at the process. She also knows how difficult it is to shut off that small but insistent voice inside that tells you to quit. Through *The Quick & Clean Diet* book, she tells you how to defeat that voice and succeed at gaining health while losing weight.

In a world constantly searching for that "magic pill," Dari's approach—through its step-by-step eating plan and easy-to-understand nutritional guidelines—puts you on the right track to losing weight without asking you to dramatically change your life or give up every food you love. Instead, Dari helps you find the foods you adore that just happen to be good for you.

The Quick & Clean Diet focuses on the practice of "clean eating," that is, consuming foods as close to their natural state as possible. This is a lifestyle very common to bodybuilders and celebrities with personal chefs, but one that is still new to the general public. With the Q & C plan you will learn the importance of eating "whole" foods—for example, an apple versus an apple-flavored whatever—and to say good-bye to fat-free, carb-free, and sugar-free foodstuffs. As the author of many books, I appreciate Dari's ability as an experienced reporter to digest and present dense scientific information in a clear, concise fashion that anyone can understand and incorporate into their lives. And as a doctor, I can vouch that Dari gets it right, whether she's sharing her expert research on how complex carbohydrates and good fats treat insulin resistance as you lose weight, or why starving yourself often paradoxically causes more weight gain.

And as a doctor, I can vouch that Dari gets it right, whether she's sharing her expert research on how complex carbohydrates and good fats treat insulin resistance as you lose weight or why starving yourself often paradoxically causes more weight gain.

If I were to use two words to describe The Quick & Clean Diet, they would be acceptance and awareness. Acceptance that your weight is appropriate and healthy for you instead of berating yourself for not being model-thin. Awareness as you expand your knowledge about the benefits of whole foods and the hazards of unhealthy eating. So start empowering yourself to meet your goal of being healthier and achieving your ideal weight. Dari knows what she is talking about, and if she can do it, you can too—you'll lose weight, look trim, have more energy, and live longer for it!

Mehmet Oz, MD
Professor and Vice Chair, Surgery
New York Presbyterian / Columbia Medical Center

We're Alike, You and Me

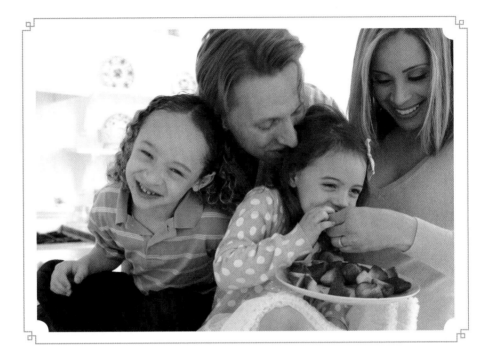

If you're reading this book, we probably have something in common. Maybe it's one (or more) of these thoughts: Losing weight is so hard! With everything going on in my life right now, I don't have time to do this! I'll start tomorrow. I don't think I'm really up to doing this right now.

Believe me, I know. I've had every one of those thoughts.

You may also have thought from time to time that you'll never be at your ideal weight. Or that people who are thin have a super-fast metabolism and you don't. Wrong! Or that skinny girls don't eat, and you love food. Wrong again!

I love food too—always have. I remember as a kid asking my mother what we were having for dinner and being either excited when it was something I loved or disappointed when it wasn't. There is no denying that food evokes emotions and memories for all of us, and I'm not trying to change that. I'm actually a culinary school graduate, and food has always been an important part of my life. I still love and look forward to all my meals—and so should you.

Do you beat yourself up because you've tried to lose weight many times and failed? Been there. Do you think you're weak because you can't control your cravings?

I know all about it.

Whatever that negative voice in your head is telling you about your inability to lose weight, I've heard it: *You'll never get there. You're a loser. You're not good enough.*

If those are the things you've been telling yourself, I'm here to say, "Stop! That's ridiculous. It doesn't have to be that way."

I got sick of that destructive voice, the negative mentality, and I bet you're sick of it too. So let's shut it off for good.

I did!

You can, once and for all, dump the negativity, the loser mentality, the guilt. And if you've been comparing yourself with others—especially celebrities—and thinking you'll never measure up, it's time to stop that too. It's okay to admire them, so long as you understand that each one of us is unique and you don't know what they did to look the way they do. It probably took (and continues to take) hard work. They don't have a magic formula any more than you and I do.

Do you get up in the morning, look in your closet, and wonder what you're going to wear because half the stuff in there doesn't fit? If so, imagine a life where you look in your closet and say, "I can wear anything I want today, because I look great in everything!"

Wouldn't it be fun to feel completely comfortable and confident wearing something crazy-sexy to a party on Saturday night? And why shouldn't you? No matter where you are in your life right now, your butt doesn't have to be that big. Your thighs don't have to be that thick, and your tummy doesn't have to look like you're wearing a tire under that T-shirt.

It can be different—and it will. I promise.

And who am I to make that promise? Well, I'm certainly not your weight loss fairy godmother. I can't wave one of my daughter's magic wands and make you instantly svelte. Although I would if I could! In reality, however, I'm a journalist and a mother—in other words, a busy working woman, just like many of you.

Some of you may know me from my work at local TV stations across America, in West Virginia, Iowa, Ohio, Dallas, or New York. Or you may know me as an anchor at the Fox News Channel. My job as a journalist and reporter is to research a topic and then deliver the information to other people in a way that is interesting, entertaining, and easy to understand.

Among the many topics I've researched and reported is the diet industry. And believe me, it is an industry. In fact, it's really big business. Millions and millions of Americans are always on a diet. We spend billions on diet books, magazines, diet programs, websites, and gyms. I've researched and reported on just about every fad diet out there. And I've probably tried every one too. But each time, like the rest of you, I've wound up right back where I started, only feeling a bit more disillusioned and defeated.

I got sick of that destructive voice, the negative mentality, and I bet you're sick of it too. So let's shut it off for good. I did!

If there's one thing I've learned, it's that fad diets are just short-term fixes. They may help you lose weight initially, but they're not sustainable, because nobody can live on cabbage soup, protein shakes, or spicy lemonade for very long.

It's as a mother, however, that my real weight issues began. Having children is the best thing I've ever done, and I adore them, but I gained nearly sixty pounds while pregnant with my two children. I had fun getting pregnant and fun gaining the weight. I loved eating all those tasty, high-calorie foods. Who wouldn't? So I did. I ate anytime, day or night. If I wanted Frosted Flakes at midnight, I ate them. Buffalo wings for breakfast, no problem! Chicken parm, barbecued ribs, guacamole, quesadillas—if I wanted it, I ate it. And I never looked back, or forward for that matter. After all, I was growing a baby.

Can you say consequences? I'm not looking for sympathy, but there I was, week thirty-eight, at the doctor's office, soon to have a son. I was on cloud nine until the nurse put me on the scale. Whoa. I had gained fifty-seven pounds, and she had my pre-pregnancy weight in her chart to prove it. I told myself I couldn't deal with this now. I had to focus on the baby.

During my last few weeks anchoring on the Fox News Channel, I was experiencing such intense lower-back pain that I could barely walk the halls or sit at the anchor desk. I remember doing news updates during *The O'Reilly Factor* while leaning forward and practically gritting my teeth. Then my doctor put me on bed rest for six weeks. It was a difficult time, but Tate's Chocolate Chip Walnut Cookies got me through.

On April 25, 2005, I had a fabulous eight-and-a-half-pound baby boy. Despite some complications all was right with the world. I was blissful.

It was the same when my baby girl was born on August 5, 2007. But each time, after focusing on my newborns for a few weeks, reality set in. I was a television anchor who had a lot of weight to lose before returning to work. With my son, I had four months to do it. With my daughter, just six weeks! It didn't happen either time. I tried. I really tried, but I failed miserably.

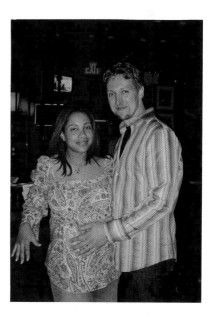

The pressure was enormous; viewers can be extremely critical, particularly on the Internet. Some plainly asked on Facebook, "When are you going to lose the baby gut?" In a chat room, somebody wrote, "It's a shame what happened to Dari. I guess sexy is now a fatty." I tried not to look at that stuff, but when it's on your Facebook wall, it's almost impossible to ignore. I felt sorry for myself, even as I frantically tried new diets. I'd have a good week or two, followed by three rebellious ones during which I ate anything I wanted. It was disastrous for my metabolism, and even worse mentally, because I was quickly developing a defeatist attitude. I thought I'd never figure this out.

I wish I could say there was one defining moment when everything changed, but it didn't happen that way. I didn't climb a mountain and suddenly see the light. Instead I started watching the HBO series *True Blood*. I remember seeing lead actress Anna Paquin prancing around the local bar, Merlotte's, in short shorts, and thinking *I used to look like that—when I was twenty-five! Why can't I look like that again, or at least close to it?* In that moment I resolved to do whatever I could to look and feel young and healthy again.

The first thing I did was Google Anna Paquin. Confirmed. She does have a great body. Then, while I working out one day, I told my trainer about my Paquin moment and, to my surprise, she told me that she actually knew all about Anna's regime because she and her husband trained her when she was in New York. What my trainer told me was that Anna Paquin, like many actresses, follows a strict diet of clean eating. That's how she stays so lean and toned.

I was intrigued—clean eating? It sounded good to me, so I immediately put on my journalist hat and began to read everything I could about clean eating. Most of what I found was in bodybuilding-oriented websites and publications. Clean eating, I discovered, is simply about eating whole, unprocessed foods, including lean protein, complex carbohydrates, and good fats. (I'll explain exactly what those terms mean in chapter 1.) I also learned that if I wanted to shell out hundreds of dollars for home-delivered meals I could easily eat clean. Or I could hire a personal chef. But those weren't realistic options for me.

I do, however, know how to cook. As I've said, I actually went to culinary school. Still, between two small children and a demanding job, I don't have a lot of time to spend in the kitchen. I needed to come up with recipes that were both quick and clean—and that also tasted good. And that's what I did.

I developed my own Quick & Clean Diet. It's helped me meet my weight loss and maintenance needs, and the recipes are delicious. It's worked so well for me that I decided I had to share it, which is why I'm writing this book.

The Quick & Clean Diet is about more than just losing weight. Yes, this back-to-basics, no-nonsense weight loss and maintenance program will make you skinny, but it will also increase your energy, and, most important, it will ensure that you enjoy lifelong good health.

It's also simple to understand and easy to remember. If I could do it, so can you. All you have to do is follow the plan. I'm sure you've followed diets before, but mine is different. Most conventional diets

We're Alike, You and Me

give you a strict program to follow for a certain period of time during which you *will* lose weight, and then you're on your own. If you talk to many people who have successfully shed pounds, they will tell you that losing weight is the easy part. The real battle comes when you're trying to keep it off. That's because most diets sell you the hype of a brand-new, revolutionary program that will whip the weight off you, and many of us, because we're so anxious to get skinny, say "Sign me up!" without considering an exit plan. Well, fear not, the Quick & Clean Diet has an exit plan, along with a beginning and a middle. You won't be abandoned here.

Truthfully, I'm not crazy about the word *diet*. It's a tricky word because it can produce strange emotions. For one, it can make you feel anxious and restricted. Or it can give you an unrealistic sense of excitement by offering what appears to be a quick fix for a long-standing problem. So do me a favor: Try not to focus too much on the word diet in this book's title. Try to think of it as a structured lifestyle plan with certain guidelines that will help you achieve your weight loss and maintenance goals. Structure is important when you're trying to make a big change. I just know from experience that if you focus too much on dieting, you may sabotage yourself. Instead think of it as a process of retraining your mind and body about food. See it as the beginning of your new life—one that will have good days and days when you will have to work harder. But above all, think of it as a commitment to being the best you can be.

*No one can make you
feel inferior without
your consent.*

—Eleanor Roosevelt

PART ONE

Clean Eating— How, What, and Why

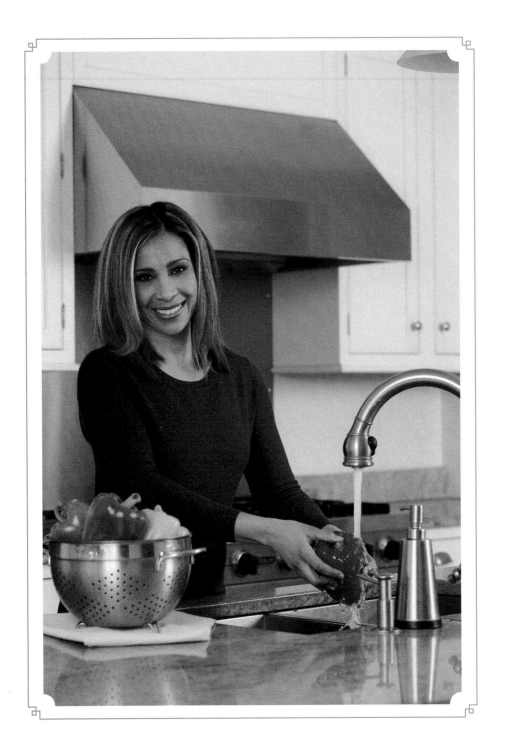

One

What It Means

If you lead a sedentary, fast-food-laden lifestyle—meaning that you spend most of your time sitting, whether at work or home, and scarfing down a drive-through lunch or dinner—you are not alone. In fact, this way of life is not only a nationwide problem, it's becoming a worldwide epidemic. As corporations continue to export tasty, processed, sugary, fatty foods to countries all over the world, millions of people face the prospect of obesity. As a reporter, I'm telling you, as long as there are billions of dollars in profits available, there is no reason for companies to stop producing food that is guaranteed to make you unhealthy and fat.

That's why what you eat is up to you. You must put your foot down. You need to begin to regulate your own behavior by turning away from what you've come to know as fast and satisfying and start to reach for foods that will actually nourish you. Do this, and skinny will be the by-product. But your first concern should always be your health.

So how do you get there?

You go clean.

Clean eating means eating foods that are processed minimally, if at all. It means consuming foods closest to their natural state. You won't find any pre-packaged, heavily processed, refined, or fast foods here. By avoiding those foods, you allow your body to rid itself of toxins and flush out unnecessary fat.

When you can, you'll be eating fruits and vegetables straight from your local market, a farmers' market, or, if possible, your own garden. No fake flavors allowed. Eat an apple, not something apple-flavored. No ingredients that you can't pronounce.

The Quick & Clean Diet is not about cutting out carbs; it's about avoiding starchy, sugary carbs. It's not about going fat-free. It's about choosing good fats. And it's about eating plenty of lean proteins, including chicken, turkey, and fish—even shrimp or tofu if you choose—while avoiding those that are high in artery-clogging saturated animal fats.

Lean Proteins Keep You Lean

When we think of protein, we generally think of meat, poultry, and fish. But there is also protein in beans, dairy, eggs, soy, and quinoa, which is a grain. In fact, soy (as in tofu) and quinoa are the only two vegetarian sources of complete protein, meaning that they provide all of the essential amino acids your body needs but can't make for itself.

Animal sources all provide complete protein, but most meat protein also comes with quite a lot of fat, and it's saturated fat, which is not very good for your heart. Chicken and turkey (particularly the white meat) have a lot less fat, especially if you remove the skin, where most of the fat is stored. And fish has omega-3 fatty acids, which your body requires. Omega-3s are polyunsaturated fats that can actually help to lower blood cholesterol and triglyceride levels and reduce your risk of heart diseases.

On the Quick & Clean Diet, you'll eat plenty of lean protein.

Fats: The Good, the Bad, and the Really Ugly

Aside from omega-3 fatty acids, the other "good fats" are monounsaturated. They are the fats that remain liquid at room temperature, which means that you probably think of them as oils. Olive oil is likely the monounsaturated fat we use most frequently, but others include canola and peanut oils. Many nuts, as well as avocados, olives, and pumpkin seeds, also contain monounsaturated fats.

On a personal note . . .
When I'm craving a little butter, I have it!
Forget the fake stuff.

Although in terms of calories, fat is fat, and all fat has 9 calories per gram—more than twice as many as either protein or carbs—your

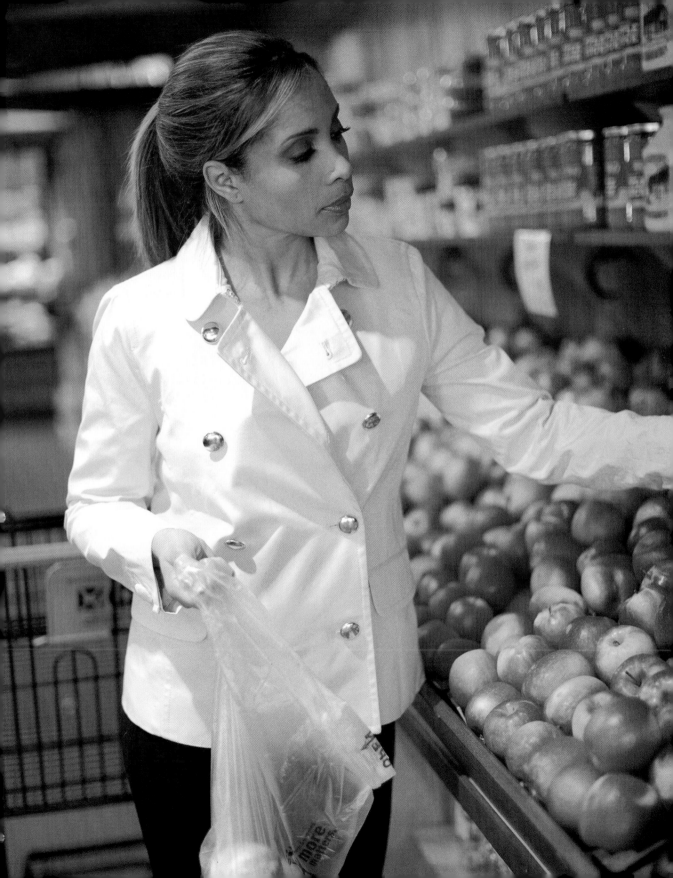

body needs fat to function, and unsaturated fats, consumed in moderation, are considered to be heart-healthy. In fact, consumption of olive oil is one reason why the diet naturally followed by people who live near the Mediterranean is considered to be so good.

Saturated fats, as I've said, are those found mainly in meat, poultry skin, eggs, and full-fat dairy products, and are known to raise LDL ("bad") cholesterol.

Trans fats are the most evil. Why? Not only because many studies have shown that they increase your LDL (bad) cholesterol, thereby increasing your risk for cardiovascular disease, but also because they are man-made. That's right: Trans fats are made by partially hydrogenating perfectly healthy vegetable oils so that they remain solid at lower temperatures, thereby helping to increase the shelf life of baked goods and many snack foods. Initially trans fats were also used to keep stick margarines solid and spreadable. Unlike animal fat (from which butter is made), vegetable oils (used to make margarine) do not solidify when cold, so the vegetable oil was partially hydrogenated to get it to solidify. Now, however, many margarines are made without trans fats. So if you use it, be sure to read the label. And any time you see the words *hydrogenated* or *partially hydrogenated* on any food package, put it back on the shelf and walk away.

Not All Carbs Are Created Equal

The truth is, carbohydrates tend to get a bad rap. That's because when people think of carbs, they immediately think about starch and sugar. But the fact is, all fruits and vegetables contain carbohydrates.

What are generally called simple carbs are, well, simply sugar. It's what's in your sugar bowl, in candy, cookies, cake, ice cream, soda, and syrups. The problem with simple carbs is that they have a lot of calories and virtually no nutritional value. They are also digested very quickly so that they give you a quick energy boost (not to mention a sweet treat) and then cause your blood sugar to drop rapidly so that you're left feeling let down and craving more. (I'll be talking much more about blood sugar levels and how they affect your weight and overall health in chapter 2.) On the Quick & Clean Diet, you'll be avoiding simple carbs.

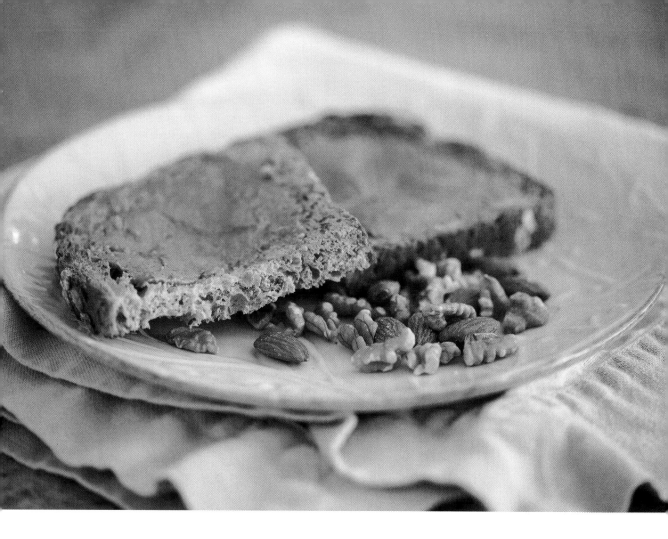

Beyond the rise and fall in blood sugar, however, studies are beginning to show that sugar is actually addictive. Researchers at Princeton University found that rats fed diets high in sugar experienced changes in the brain similar to those associated with people who abuse drugs like cocaine and heroin. When they were deprived of sugar, the rats got "the shakes"—a symptom generally associated with withdrawal from drugs or alcohol.

In addition, Dr. Robert Lustig and his colleagues at the University of California–San Francisco have studied the effects of sugar on brain chemistry and concluded that consuming sugar causes us to simultaneously feel hungry and store fat. Furthermore, these researchers confirmed that sugar is addictive in much the same way as drugs and alcohol.

That sounds pretty scary to me!

Complex carbs are basically starch—that is, a bunch of sugar molecules strung together—which is turned into glucose (sugar) when we digest it. All kinds of grains, as well as potatoes, rice, and beans, are complex carbohydrates. Grains are used to make pasta, breads, and cereals, and the kinds of grains that are used generally determine how quickly they turn to sugar after you eat them. Whole grains are the least processed and therefore take the longest to digest, meaning that they don't cause your blood sugar to spike and drop as quickly as more highly processed grains. So whole wheat bread is better than white bread; whole wheat pasta is better than white pasta; and whole grain cereals are better than those that have been flaked or puffed (and certainly better than those that have been presweetened).

But what about fruits and vegetables? Well, all fruits are basically fructose (fruit sugar), which your body turns into glucose. And all vegetables contain some carbohydrates. Some fruits (such as bananas) and vegetables (such as corn) are "starchier" than others. But all fruits and vegetables also contain important nutrients, and they all contain substantial amounts of fiber.

Fiber is important for a couple of reasons. First of all, it takes longer for your body to process foods that contain a lot of fiber, which means that they turn to sugar much more slowly and don't cause your blood sugar to spike. And second, fiber is indigestible, so it helps you to feel full without adding calories to your meal.

When you read about the three stages of the Quick & Clean Diet in part 2, you'll see that the kinds of carbs you're allowed to eat in Stage One (the cleansing and jump-starting stage) are quite restricted. Then, as you move to Stage Two and Stage Three, more and more carbs will be included so that your new way of eating becomes easily sustainable for the rest of your life.

What You Need to Know about the Glycemic Index

If you've been on any kind of diet in the last decade or so, you've no doubt heard about the glycemic index. And you probably know that consuming foods with a low glycemic index rating is "good," while

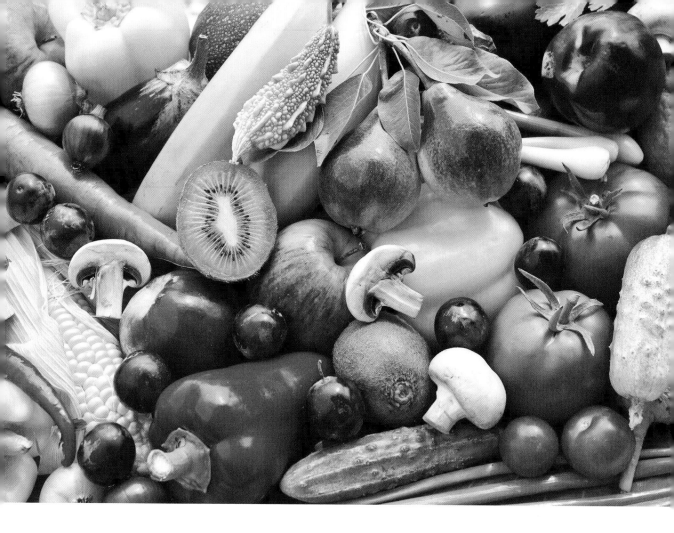

foods high on the glycemic index are "bad." But do you actually know what all that means?

Actually, the glycemic index is a measure of the degree to which foods that contain carbohydrates raise your blood sugar. Glucose—that is, pure sugar—is rated 100, and all other foods are rated relative to that. So basically, simple carbs and starchy complex carbs are listed highest on the index while most vegetables (including all the leafy greens) and many fruits (such as blueberries, blackberries, and strawberries) are lower.

The carbs you'll eat on this diet are all relatively low on the glycemic index.

How It's Going to Work

In part 2 I'll give you a step-by-step guide with food lists and meal plans, but before you begin you'd probably like to know what you're signing up for. I know I would. So here's a quick overview.

The Quick & Clean Diet is, as I've said, divided into three stages.

STAGE ONE

High Motivation is designed to detox your system from all the bad stuff you've probably been putting in your body, stabilize your blood sugar, kill your cravings, and jump-start your weight loss. It is definitely the most restrictive stage, but it's only for fourteen days and the rewards you'll see in terms of looser clothes, greater energy, and a sharper mind will be well worth the effort. By the time it's over, a switch in your brain will have flipped, the lightbulb will go on, and you'll be thinking, *Wow, I really like what's happening here.*

> *On a personal note . . .*
>
> It's true—this part isn't easy. But dig in deep. I did! You'll be very pleased with yourself when you see the results.

STAGE TWO

Grounding is when you'll start to add a wider variety of foods to your meal plan. You'll lose about two pounds a week—although everyone is different, so you may lose more or less—and your body will continue to change in the way it responds to food. Soon you'll find that you no longer long for those sweet and simple carbs. Instead you'll actually crave the clean, whole foods that give your body more energy and your brain more clarity. You may not even have realized how fuzzy and sluggish you used to feel so much of the time. That was all a part of the blood sugar highs and lows that are no longer a part of your life.

Stability: You'll stay on the Grounding Stage until you reach your goal weight and then move on to Stability. Here you will eat an even wider variety of foods and be more motivated than ever to maintain your new slim and sexy figure.

The goal, of course, is to maintain good health and stable eating habits. Realistically, however, this may be challenging at times. But now that you know what to do and how to do it, if you do fall off the horse, so to speak, during the holidays or when you're on vacation, you'll be able to get right back on by returning to the High Motivation Stage for a week or two before the situation gets out of hand.

But before we get all excited about looking fabulous (you will!), we need to talk about why it's so important to be at your proper weight.

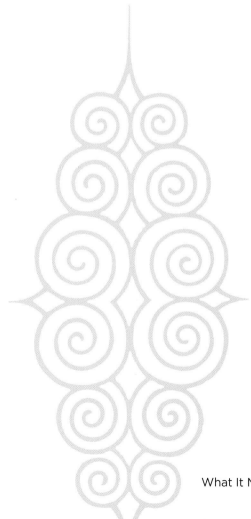

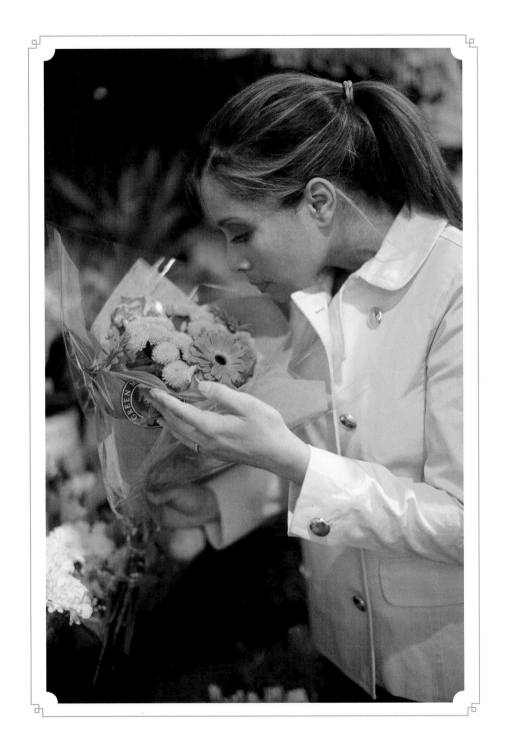

Two

It's Really All about Health

You're probably thinking you just want to look better. I get it. My primary motivation for losing weight was also the mirror. But losing those extra pounds will make you feel better, and it will have significant long-term benefits for your overall health. One of the worst things about being overweight and out of shape is the way you feel on a day-to-day basis. Lethargy, lack of motivation and focus, and insomnia are common symptoms, and that's not even the serious stuff. You may not even realize that you feel horrible, because you're so used to it, but believe me, this is no way to live. You deserve to feel better. And you certainly deserve to live a long, healthy life.

I certainly don't claim to be a health care professional, and I don't mean to be giving you medical advice. But I do want to share some of the most important information I've gathered about the more serious health risks associated with being overweight.

Heart Disease and Diabetes

According to the American Heart Association, simply being 20 percent above your ideal weight, independent of any other risk factors, increases your risk for heart disease, stroke, high blood pressure, diabetes, and more.

The groundbreaking Framingham Heart Study, which has been following a cohort of 5,209 men and women from Framingham, Massachusetts, since 1948, did a twenty-six-year follow-up and found that the relative weight of the participants upon entering the study was predictive of their developing cardiovascular disease and also that weight gain after young adulthood increased the risk of heart disease.

In 1997 a Statement for Healthcare Professionals issued by the Nutrition Committee of the American Heart Association pointed out that, in addition to obesity being an independent risk factor for coronary heart disease, obese people were more likely to have high blood pressure, lower levels of HDL (good) cholesterol, insulin resistance, and Type 2 diabetes, all of which are also associated with heart disease.

Although results have varied, the majority of scientific studies find that reducing your dietary intake of trans fats (found most often in commercial baked goods, stick margarine, snack foods, chips, and frozen dinners) and saturated fats (from fatty meats and animal products like butter, full-fat milk, and cream) reduces your risk of developing heart disease. And reducing your intake of dietary fat will also lead to weight loss.

What may not be so immediately apparent, however, is how your blood sugar is related to heart health, but it is. A study conducted in Norfolk, England, and published in the *Annals of Internal Medicine* followed 4,662 men and 5,570 women from 1995 to 1997 and found that the participants' average blood glucose levels were directly related to their incidence of cardiovascular disease and death. And according to the National Institutes of Health, adults with diabetes are two to four times more likely to have heart disease or suffer a stroke than those who don't have diabetes. About 65 percent of people with diabetes die from heart disease and stroke.

Diabetic Care Services states on their website that 80 to 90 percent of people who are diagnosed with Type 2 diabetes are also diagnosed as obese. The relationship between weight and diabetes is complicated, but the fact is that being overweight adversely affects your body's ability to control blood sugar levels, leading to what is called insulin resistance. When you consume foods that are metabolized as glucose (that is, any kind of sugar or starch), your pancreas releases insulin to remove the excess glucose from your bloodstream in order to keep your blood sugar level. Being insulin-resistant means that your body needs to make more and more insulin just to do its job. When the pancreas is no longer able to keep up with the demand for insulin, your blood sugar levels rise, which, over time, can lead to diabetes.

Weight Is Also Linked with Cancer

The National Cancer Institute states that excess weight and obesity have been linked to an increased risk for various types of cancer, particularly breast and endometrial cancer in women, colorectal cancer particularly in men, and kidney, esophageal, gallbladder, and thyroid cancer in both men and women. For breast and endometrial cancer, the increased risk seems to be linked to the high levels of estrogen produced by fat tissue. For colorectal cancer there appears to be a link particularly with excess abdominal fat. And for all types of cancer, researchers believe that insulin resistance also plays a role.

Other Health Issues

Nonalcoholic fatty liver disease is just what it sounds like—too much fat in the liver that isn't caused by drinking alcohol but may be the result of eating too many marbled steaks, too much fried food, or too much ice cream—to name just a few of the many sources of fat in the average American diet. And this too is linked to insulin resistance. Although we tend to think of the role insulin plays in the regulation of blood sugar, it is also a key factor in the way we metabolize fat. Insulin triggers the secretion of an enzyme that increases the uptake of fat from the bloodstream for storage in various cells, including the liver. So the more insulin there is in your blood, the more fat your body will store, leading to an increased accumulation of fat in the liver. (This, by the way, was the basic premise of the Atkins diet: Your body only stores fat in the presence of insulin, and you only produce insulin in the presence of glucose. So if you don't eat carbs, you don't produce insulin, and, therefore, you don't store fat.)

Studies have shown that as your BMI or body mass index (which expresses the ratio of your weight in relation to your height) increases, so does the amount of fat in your liver.

On a personal note . . .

When I first learned about all of these health concerns, it seemed intimidating. But I realized that I was happy to know it because it made me understand the importance of maintaining a healthy weight.

Being overweight or obese also puts you at higher risk for developing gallstones. The gallbladder stores bile, which is secreted by the liver, and releases it as needed to help with the digestion of fat. Gallstones are made primarily of cholesterol, and obese people tend to have higher levels of cholesterol than lean people. These higher cholesterol levels lead to the production of bile that contains more cholesterol than can be dissolved, and when that happens, it can lead to the formation of gallstones.

According to the US surgeon general, being overweight or obese is also known to be associated with high blood pressure (often called the silent killer), which is also the leading cause of stroke. In fact, high blood pressure is twice as common among obese people as it is among those who are a healthy weight.

Obesity also increases your risk for developing arthritis and asthma, and for experiencing sleep apnea, all of which can be painful, debilitating, and in some cases life threatening.

The Good News

I know, just thinking about how your weight may be affecting your health can be pretty scary. But I do want you to understand that what you're going to be doing to reduce your waistline will also significantly increase your chances of being healthier for years to come.

And the good news is that the National Heart, Lung, and Blood Institute of the National Institutes of Health has indicated that a loss of just 5 to 10 percent of your body weight over a period of six months can reduce your risk for all these diseases. For a 200-pound man, that means a loss of just 10 to 20 pounds; for a 150-pound woman, it's 7 ½ to 15 pounds. You don't need a calculator to figure it out. Just weigh yourself and move the decimal point one place to the left: That's 10 percent. Now divide that number in half and you have 5 percent.

And maintaining a loss of just that amount is more beneficial than losing even more and regaining it. Maintaining weight loss is key, and the Quick & Clean Diet is set up to make sure you are able do that.

First of all, eating all those low-glycemic vegetables and fruits will keep your blood sugar level, which means that you won't be overproducing insulin or experiencing all the health complications that this can cause. And sticking with lean proteins means that you'll avoid the saturated and trans fats that can increase your levels of LDL (bad cholesterol), which sticks to and clogs up the arteries that feed your heart and your brain, and decrease good (HDL) cholesterol, which, at high levels, seems to protect against heart disease.

So the Quick & Clean Diet isn't just about getting into your skinny jeans, although it will certainly help you do that. It's also about making sure that you're skinny and *healthy*, because, really, what could be more important than your health? I know that's a cliché, but the reason certain sayings have become clichés in the first place is that they are so true!

Now that you know what the Quick & Clean Diet will do for you, it's time to learn the 6 simple rules that will ensure you get the job done.

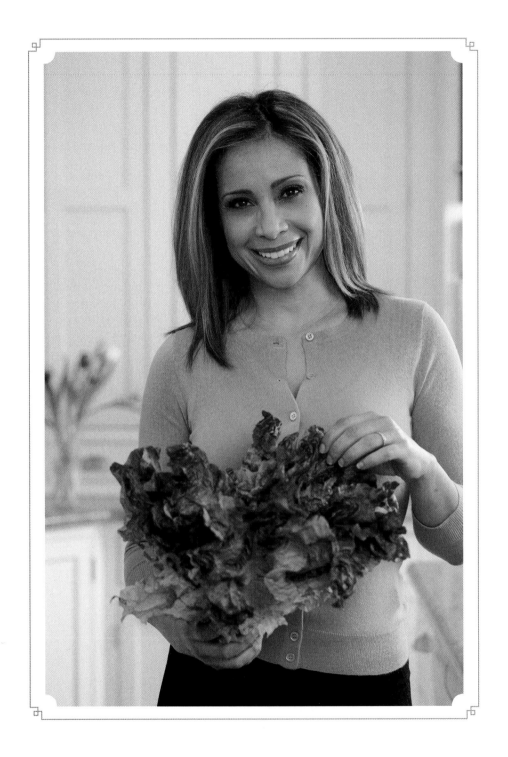

Three

Get the SKINNY— The 6 Commandments of Going Quick & Clean

Believe me, I'm not trying to be God, and I certainly can't "command" you to do or not do anything. But I do think that having a few simple rules is the best way to stay on track no matter what you're trying to achieve. Too many rules and it becomes too hard to stick to; too few and it's also hard, because you're not sure what you're supposed to be doing.

So I've come up with 6 simple rules that are easy to remember and that will keep you on the straight and narrow as you follow the path I've blazed to get you to Destination Skinny.

First Commandment: Eat foods that are as close as possible to their natural state.

We've gotten away from eating foods the way God made them, as in an actual orange or apple. Although the "whole foods" movement is catching on slowly, for a long time it seemed that you could get something apple- or orange-flavored a lot more easily than you could an apple or an orange. Go to Starbucks and ask for a cranberry-, banana-, or pumpkin-flavored latte and you got it. No problem! And have you noticed that you can get practically any fruit-flavored vodka you want? Orange, lemon, pear, pineapple, peach, strawberry, raspberry, coconut, apple, watermelon . . . Did I miss one? Is there a chocolate-flavored vodka? Of course there is!

You know we're on the wrong path when it's easier to buy fruit-flavored liquor or coffee than it is to find an apple at a convenience store or a coffee shop,

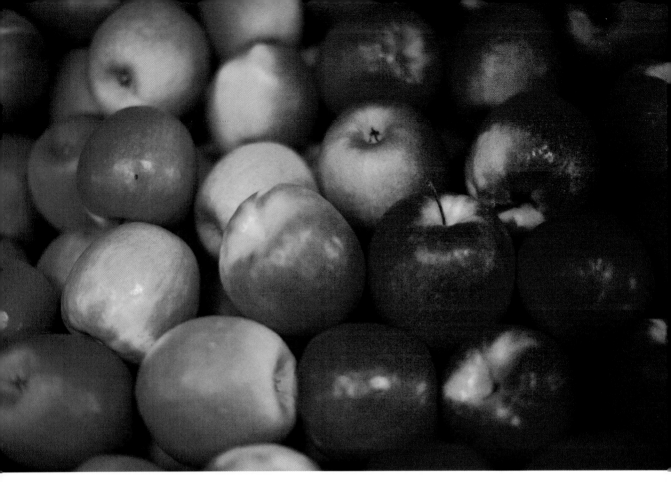

Foods in their most natural state provide the most nutrition, and remember, that's why you're eating. I'm sure that when you shop for other things, you want to get the best quality for the least amount of money. And it shouldn't be any different for food. You should be looking for the most flavor and the most nutrients for the fewest chemicals and calories.

Have you ever heard the term *energy-dense* with relation to food? Do you know what it means? I didn't when I started researching clean eating. In fact, I thought it sounded like something pretty good—maybe foods that give you a lot of energy. But when I looked it up, I discovered that energy-dense foods are those that have a lot of calories packed into a small amount of food. A calorie is a unit of energy, so when you read or hear about how many calories you "burn" when you're engaging in some particular kind of activity like walking, bike riding, or swimming for a particular length of time, what that really means is how much *energy* it takes. When foods are low-energy-dense, it means you can eat more of them because they have fewer calories. Interestingly, a study conducted by members of the nutrition department at Pennsylvania State University found that when people were fed diets that varied in energy density and could eat as much as they wanted, they ate the same quantity of food by weight no matter how energy-dense the food. What this means is that if you're consuming foods with a low energy density, you can eat until you're satisfied and not pay the high-calorie price.

{ *On a personal note . . .*

I've learned to fill up on steamed broccoli or spinach with lemon. Nutrient-dense foods have become the most important part of my dinner. }

What we should be looking for is foods—like leafy green vegetables, white-meat chicken, and fish—that have low energy density but are nutrient-dense, meaning that they are rich in nutrients compared with their calorie content. Those are mainly foods that are in their natural state and not packed with added sugar or other ingredients that don't have any nutritional value.

Second Commandment: Feed your body every three hours.

When most of us thing of losing weight, we think about starving. I know I did. And on previous diets I really was hungry all the time. But not on the Quick & Clean Diet. Just the opposite; I *want* you to eat something every three hours. I *never* want you to be starving. That's why, in chapter 14, I'll be providing a wide variety of recipes and choices for all three meals as well as Quick & Clean snacks.

Some diet gurus advocate eating several small meals throughout the day, and that works just fine for many people. But I like to be more traditional, focusing on three main meals and two snacks. Not only does that keep me more in tune with the way most people eat, but thinking of those in-between meals as snacks also helps me to stick to the program by keeping me satisfied while reminding me not to overeat.

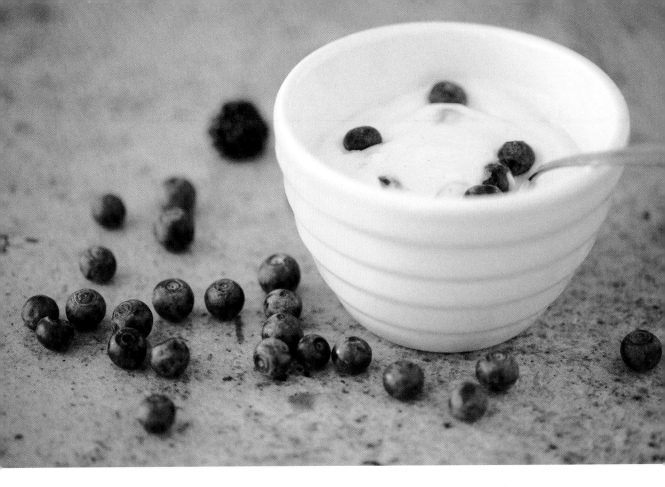

Those snacks are important psychologically too, because if you know you're not "allowed" to eat until the next mealtime all you can think about is how much longer you have to wait and what you're going to eat when you do. In other words, all you think about is food. And if you let yourself get to the point where you think you're hungry enough to eat a horse, there's a really good chance that, when you finally do sit down to eat, you'll grab everything in sight.

For years I felt that if my stomach was growling, it meant that I was being successful on my diet. If I was on a diet, I was *supposed* to be hungry. Not so! Maybe you can sustain being hungry for a few days or even a few weeks, but being hungry is simply not sustainable for long, and your goal, after all, is to change your eating habits for life.

I now know that, almost inevitably, I *will* be hungry before dinner, and it's okay to eat something, as long as it's the right something. So I'm prepared. In chapter 14 I'll give you a number of snack choices you can always have on hand that will keep you satisfied until your next mealtime without sabotaging all the good work you've already done.

Aside from the psychological advantage of knowing that you don't have to go all the way from breakfast to lunch or lunch to dinner without eating anything, there are some sound scientific reasons for never getting to the point where you're running on empty. For one thing, your blood sugar will have dropped and your brain will be demanding a quick fix, which usually means heading for the nearest candy or soda machine.

Willpower is great, but it will take you only so far. When your blood sugar hits a low point, you're not thinking clearly, you're cranky, your energy is low, and willpower just isn't going to do it for you. Having a snack prevents that from happening, and I also find that it makes me more productive and a lot more pleasant to be around.

But there's yet another reason for never letting your body wonder where its next meal is coming from.

Back in the days when our ancestors were hunter-gatherers, it really was feast or famine, and they could never be sure when they'd be eating again. So the people who ate the most—and therefore stored the most fat—were the most likely to survive, because they could burn that fat for energy when food was scarce.

Now, of course, at least in the developed world, our next meal is never more than a supermarket or a take-out menu away, but our bodies are still operating on the principle that if they haven't been fueled in a while, there's probably a famine and they need to go into conservation mode. Your metabolism then automatically slows down, and you also tend to become more sluggish and sedentary (the better to conserve your energy stores). What that means if you're trying to lose weight is that your body is working against you instead of with you. Instead of increasing your metabolic rate and burning more calories faster, you're doing exactly the opposite!

Knowing that, it should also be clear that you must *never* skip a meal. We've all done it—decided we're going to skip breakfast and/or lunch and "save up" our calories for dinner. Don't do it! And, above all, *don't skip breakfast.* A study done of participants in the National Weight Control Registry (which includes three thousand individuals who have successfully lost at least thirty pounds and maintained the loss for at least one year) found that 80 percent of those in the study ate breakfast every day as part of their weight maintenance routine.

I've heard people say that they don't like breakfast or they don't have time to eat it. On the Quick & Clean Diet, there is no room for those excuses. I provide recipes for smoothies you can whip up in a minute and drink while you're dressing. I also provide a wide variety of options so that there's sure to be something for everyone's taste. Even on the most restrictive stage of the diet, you can have bacon and eggs if that's what you want. Or how about a breakfast quiche? And when you get to Stage Two, there's a recipe for pancakes. Some days you'll be feeling more adventurous or have more time than others. Those are the days when you can try new things or spend more time preparing. And when you just want something quick and comforting, there will be choices for those days as well.

Third Commandment: Include lean protein, complex carbohydrates, and friendly fats in every meal.

Your body needs all the major nutrients to stay healthy, and you need them to feel satisfied.

Unless you have kidney or liver disease, you've probably never been on a low-protein diet. And if you do have those health issues, I'm assuming you're under the care of a doctor who is monitoring your diet and making sure you get adequate protein from vegetarian sources. I am certainly not equipped and would never attempt to offer that kind of advice. But if you're reasonably healthy, you should get some protein at every meal, because your body requires it just to

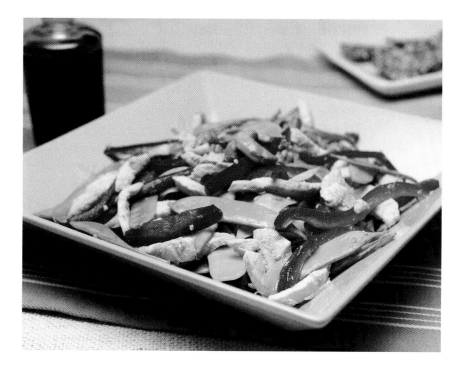

stay alive. Protein, as I've already said, provides essential amino acids that you must get from food sources.

But from a weight loss perspective, protein does something else important as well—it keeps you feeling fuller longer. In fact, a study published in *The American Journal of Clinical Nutrition* reported that people felt less hunger and experienced greater weight loss when they increased their protein intake to 30 percent of their total diet. And another study published in the journal *Appetite* found that a high-protein afternoon snack delayed the request for dinner by sixty minutes, far longer than either a high-carb or a high-fat snack.

Finally, protein has been found to reduce appetite, which means, of course, that it helps you feel less hungry. While the mechanism for doing this isn't entirely clear, one theory is that protein contains tryptophan, an essential amino acid that is a precursor to the production of serotonin, which is a neurotransmitter responsible for regulating mood, appetite, and sleep. So eating protein may increase serotonin levels, causing us to feel more satisfied.

Do you remember the fen-phen diet pill craze of the 1990s? Do you know how it worked? In fact, it was a combination of two medications working synergistically. One of those medications, fenfluramine, increases the levels of serotonin available for the body to use, which tricks the body into feeling fuller and decreasing your appetite. The other drug, phentermine, is similar to an amphetamine (aka speed). The problem is that in addition to speeding up your metabolism, it also increases your blood pressure, speeds up your heart rate, and causes palpitations. I don't know about you, but I'd rather get my feelings of satiety and energy from healthy, nutritious food. And I certainly don't want to put myself as risk for hypertension or heart problems in order to reduce my waist size.

So what about carbs? First of all, your body craves them, and second, it needs them to be healthy. All carbohydrates are plant-based foods, and all plant-based foods contain carbohydrates—often with some protein and sometimes also with some good, healthy fat.

We've already talked about the difference between simple and complex carbs—that is, between sugary, starchy carbs (baked goods, white bread, pasta, and the like) that quickly turn to glucose in your body, and those such as spinach, broccoli, artichokes, bell peppers, and onions that you digest more slowly. On the Quick & Clean Diet, you'll be eating plenty of low-glycemic vegetables and fruits that help to fill you up without filling you out. In fact, most vegetables are so low in calories that you can eat as much of them as you want. And the new "food plate" issued by the US Department of Agriculture in 2011 shows that fully half the plate should be filled with fruits and vegetables.

Fruits and vegetables also contain large quantities of phytonutrients—chemical compounds that can only be found in plant foods and that are generally filled with antioxidants, which protect our cells from the damage that leads to aging and disease.

And finally there are fats. As with both protein and carbs, it's a question of how much and what kind of fats you are eating. In terms of weight control, all fat has 9 calories per gram (as opposed to just over 4 calories per gram for both protein and carbs). So eating too much of any kind of fat can cause calories to add up. But aside from calorie content, as we've already discussed, too much saturated fat and virtually all trans fat is bad for your health.

On the other hand, healthy fats, including olive oil and safflower oil, are necessary for building and maintaining cellular integrity, and for proper brain function. In fact, our brain is composed of 60 percent fat! But probably the most exciting thing I learned while researching the Quick & Clean Diet is that consuming the right kind of fat can actually help us to burn fat faster. Again, as with the information on clean eating, I learned about this first from bodybuilding websites. Here's how it works: Omega-3 fatty acids (see chapter 1) help the body respond better to a hormone called leptin—often called the "I'm full" hormone—secreted by fat tissue, which signals your brain that you're full. So the more in tune your brain is to these messages, the better appetite control you will have.

In addition, if you deprive your body of dietary fat (and so long as you're consuming carbs to provide energy), it will do everything in its power to hang on to the fat it's got. Remember that back in our hunter-gatherer days (where our bodies still live), he who had the most fat lived longest!

Fourth Commandment: Avoid heavily processed foods.

Processed foods, as we've discussed, are basically those that have been altered from their natural state. Not only does all that "processing" often cause them to lose much of their nutritional value (such as when the bran is removed from wheat to make white—as opposed to whole wheat—flour), but also, in many cases, unhealthy ingredients are added for texture, color, shelf life, or to make the food more palatable. The Food and Drug Administration (FDA) allows the use of all these additives in the production, processing, treatment, packaging, transportation, or storage of food. I suppose they are necessary if you are going to buy foods so altered from their original state that they need

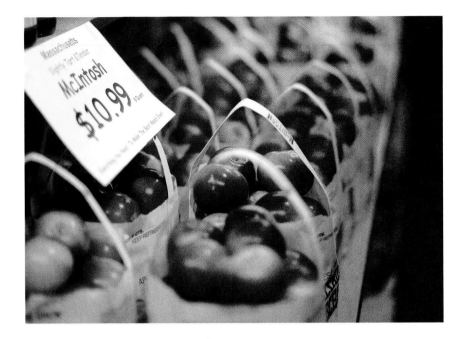

flavor and color put back into them, or if they were made in a factory six months ago and are expected to last for several weeks or even months in the grocery store or your pantry. Sound appealing? Not to me! Do you really want *gum* in your salad dressing? Xanthan gum is commonly used in salad dressings, chocolate pudding, ice cream, and other rich and creamy factory-produced foods. I don't know about you, but if I'm going to have gum, I want to chew it and then spit it out!

Still, the FDA argues that:

- Emulsifiers, stabilizers, and thickeners give foods the texture and consistency people want.

- Texturizers appeal to your sense of taste and make foods more enjoyable.

- Artificial coloring makes foods more inviting to look at.

- Artificial flavoring gives foods a more intense identity.

- A variety of additives extend the shelf-life of packaged foods.

So let me ask you this—do you really want to consume foods that contain ingredients you've never heard of or can't pronounce? Here are just a few: acesulfame-K, butylated hydroxytoluene, maltitol, monosodium glutamate, olestra, potassium bromate, propyl gallate, and sodium nitrite.

Now let me tell you what they are since you've probably been eating them without even knowing it:

Acesulfame-K is an artificial sweetener found in baked goods, chewing gum, gelatin desserts, and, of course, diet soda.

Butylated hydroxytoluene (BHT) retards rancidity in oils. You can find it in breakfast cereal, chewing gum, and potato chips.

Maltitol is an artificial sweetener found in candy, chocolates, jams, and other sugar-free foods.

Monosodium glutamate (MSG) is a flavor enhancer used in soups, salad dressings, chips, frozen foods, and lots of restaurant foods. (If you're sensitive to it, it can give you a headache.)

> *On a personal note . . .*
> When you see the word processed, read "fake." Processed cheese food isn't real cheese, and it isn't real food!

Olestra (Olean) is a fat substitute found in foods like chips. (It can cause abdominal cramps and diarrhea and has been banned in the UK and Canada.)

Potassium bromate is a flour enhancer found in foods like white flour and rolls. It strengthens dough and allows it to rise higher, but studies have shown that it may be carcinogenic; it has been banned in several countries including the European Union, Canada, and China. The FDA has urged bakers to voluntarily stop using it, and California requires a warning label on products containing it.

Propyl gallate is a preservative used in vegetable oil, meat products, potato sticks, chicken soup base, and chewing gum to prevent them from turning rancid.

Sodium nitrite is used to enhance the flavor and color and to preserve cured meats such as bacon, ham, frankfurters, cold cuts, and corned beef as well as cured fish.

I've found that if you don't know what it is and you can't pronounce it, you should probably avoid it!

In addition to all the artificial additives, however, highly processed foods such as frozen dinners (even those that are called diet dinners) are often extremely high in sodium, which can cause water retention and bloating, not to mention high blood pressure, which puts you at increased risk for heart attacks and stroke. The Centers for Disease Control and Prevention states that most of us should be consuming no more than twenty-three hundred milligrams of sodium per day. However, most Americans are getting about 9.6 grams a day, or more than four times the recommended amount. And more than 75 percent of that comes from processed foods and foods we eat in restaurants.

{ *On a personal note . . .*
I try not to eat store-bought foods with ingredients I can't pronounce or that sound like a chemical. }

Speaking of processed foods, refined white sugar is about as processed as you can get. It starts out as sugarcane, from which all the fiber is eliminated by extraction; then it's spun in a centrifuge until all that's left are those lovely white crystals that falsely promise to "sweeten" your life while offering absolutely no nutritional value. (If you've already forgotten some of the bad things sugar can do to your brain and your body, take a look back at chapters 1 and 2.)

My recommendation is that you do the majority of your food shopping in the aisles around the outside of the supermarket where the fresh produce, fish, poultry, and meats are kept. Not only will you avoid temptation, but you'll also avoid stocking up on a lot of unhealthy stuff. The only things I buy now in the middle aisles of the market are whole grain pastas and cereal, wild and brown rice, and the "pantry helpers" listed in chapter 5.

Fifth Commandment: Don't obsess about calories.

I can't tell you never to count calories, because at the end of the day, if you take in more calories than you expend, you'll gain weight. If you take in fewer than you burn, you'll lose weight. That's a basic law of thermodynamics.

You burn a certain number of calories in a twenty-four-hour period just by your body performing its essential functions even when you are in a non-active state—that's called your basal (or resting) metabolic rate. It varies somewhat depending on your age, height, and weight, and you get to add some calories depending on your degree of activity. There are formulas you can find online for determining exactly how many calories you need to maintain your weight; obviously, if you consume fewer than you need, you'll lose weight. But that's all very complicated, and the good news is that obsessively counting calories isn't really necessary on the Quick & Clean Diet.

That said, I have provided for you the nutrition information for all the recipes and calories consumed each day on the fourteen-day plan. This is merely for those who either insist upon knowing how much they are consuming out of habit, or for those who require this information for medical reasons. By the way, if you have health issues that cause you to be under a doctor's care, it is imperative that you check with your doctor before even thinking about committing to any weight loss plan. The Quick & Clean Diet is about making you feel and look better, but you need to be smart and make sure it helps, not hurts, your health.

If you eat the foods on the lists I provide in the portions suggested for each stage of the diet, you will lose weight without obsessing about calories. It's really portion distortion that causes most of our problems. Research published in the *New England Journal of Medicine* has found that people who are unsuccessfully trying to lose weight tend to *underestimate* their food intake by as much as 47 percent. That's why you may find writing down what you eat each day to be helpful and eye opening: It forces you to confront your food choices. No hiding anymore! It's all right in front of you.

If you're eating fresh, whole foods, stick to the portion size I provide, and if you're buying something that comes in a package be sure to make note of how many servings the package contains. It's written right there at the top of the Nutrition Facts label, but many of us don't pay attention and assume that one package equals one serving. Not so! Don't get fooled!

Sixth Commandment: Drink lots of water.

I have friends who tell me they hate water and they just can't do this. You know what I tell them? I tell them to just suck it up. Suck, sip, drink it up, just get it down!

First of all, I don't really understand why anyone would hate water. What is there to hate about it? But beyond that, drinking a lot of water is important for everyone and absolutely essential if you want to lose weight. You've probably heard the old advice about drinking eight glasses a day; well, I drink three liters a day! That's almost a gallon, or, in terms of an eight-ounce glass, almost thirteen

On a personal note . . .

I've found that flavored waters can make all the difference when I get bored with the plain stuff.

glasses. And believe me, that alone has made a huge difference in my weight loss and how my body looks. Also, it feels great to be hydrated. You will have more energy and feel more alert.

Water helps you lose weight in many different ways. On the simplest level, it fills you up so that you're likely to be less hungry. One study published in the *Journal of the American Dietetic Association* found that people who drank water before meals ate approximately 75 fewer calories at their meal compared with those who didn't drink water. In addition, many of us tend to think we're hungry when really we're only thirsty. So if you think you're hungry, drink water; you may find that you weren't really hungry after all.

But there's more. A small study done in Germany found that drinking seventeen ounces of water raised the study subjects' metabolic rate by 30 percent, starting about ten minutes after they drank the water and peaking thirty to forty minutes later. The researchers estimated that by increasing their water consumption by a liter and a half a day, people could burn an extra 17,400 calories (representing a five-pound weight loss) in the course of a year. And that's without changing anything else in their diet or level of activity.

And finally, remember what happens when you don't eat enough? Your body thinks it's starving and holds on to those calories. Well, the same is true of water. We need water to stay alive, so if you don't drink enough, your body will start to hold on to what it's got, making you look puffy and bloated. Not a pretty picture!

So I repeat: Drink, drink, drink! And if you're one of those people who don't like the taste of water, add a squeeze of lemon, lime, or orange to make it more palatable. Or make your own flavored water (see chapter 7).

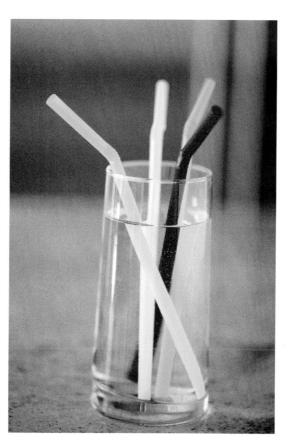

That's the skinny on eating quick and clean. Start following these 6 simple rules and I promise that you'll start to see the results within days.

To get you started, in the next chapter I'll introduce several foods that you are free to embrace. Many times when we start a new eating program, we obsess about what we *can't* eat; with the Q & C plan, however, you focus on what you *can* eat. Take a look.

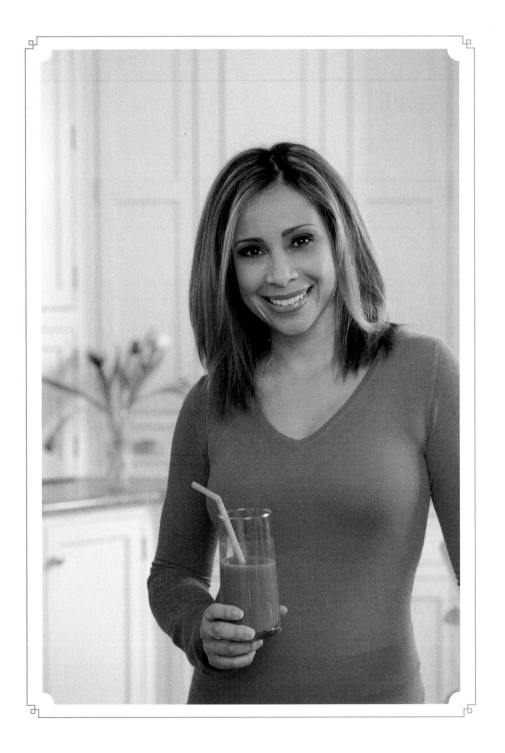

Four

Quick & Clean Foods to Love

All of these foods are about to become your new BFFs. If you've been on diets before (and most of us have), you'll probably be surprised by how much variety there is on the following lists. That's because your BFFs are *forever*, and that's a long time, so I don't want you to feel deprived.

A few of the foods I list may be restricted or not allowed during Stage One, High Motivation. But that's just two weeks—not forever. So you can look forward to welcoming them back into your life in the Grounding and Stability Stages.

Now let's take a look at everything you *can* eat when you go quick and clean. If you stick with your BFFs, you'll feel energetic, well nourished, satisfied—and never guilty.

Vegetables

Artichokes: One of my favorites, artichokes are packed with antioxidants, and I love them steamed with a dipping sauce of olive oil and lemon juice.

Arugula has eight times the calcium, five times the vitamin A, vitamin C, and vitamin K, and four times the iron as the same amount of iceberg lettuce—not to mention that it tastes amazing. Equally great in salads and on sandwiches, it's probably my favorite type of lettuce.

Asparagus: These long green stalks are not only delicious and simple to prepare, but also high in folate and a great source of potassium, fiber, thiamin, and vitamins A, B6, and C. Fabulous steamed plain or with a squeeze of lemon.

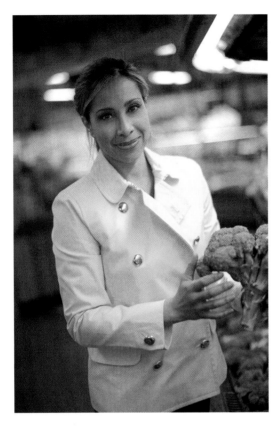

Bamboo shoots: You've probably had them in Chinese food, but bamboo adds crunch and a cornlike flavor to any salad or stir-fry. And from a health perspective, they have 2 grams of protein, 1.2 grams of fiber, and 18 percent of your daily potassium requirements in just one cup. Not bad!

Bell peppers (all colors): They come in a rainbow of gorgeous colors, and a cup of chopped bell peppers provides more than 100 percent of your daily requirements of vitamin C as well as folate, vitamin K, and a lot of fiber. Eaten raw as a snack or in salads, they pack a great crunch. Or throw them on the grill with a spritz of nonstick olive oil cooking spray and serve them as an antipasto or a side dish.

Broccoli: A dream vegetable! Broccoli is a rich source of phytochemicals (nutrients found in plant-based foods) that are known to fight cancer! It's also great for your eyes and is known to fortify your immune system. Eat it raw or steamed, with lemon and a drizzle of olive oil, or sprinkled with a little Bragg's Aminos (see chapter 5).

Brussels sprouts: These little jewels are loaded with fiber as well as antioxidants called flavonoids that have been shown to protect against certain types of cancer, and they contain more than 100 percent of your daily requirement of vitamin C. Try them steamed and drizzled with lemon and olive oil, sautéed with a bit of oil or nonstick cooking spray, or roasted. Or grate them raw into salads.

Cabbage (red or green): Along with broccoli, cauliflower, and brussels sprouts, cabbage is a cruciferous vegetable, and all cruciferous vegetables are known for their many disease-fighting and other important health benefits. Red cabbage (because of the polyphenols that provide its red color) is even higher in antioxidants than green. Have it steamed as a side; place on a plate and lay a protein over it; or grate it into coleslaw.

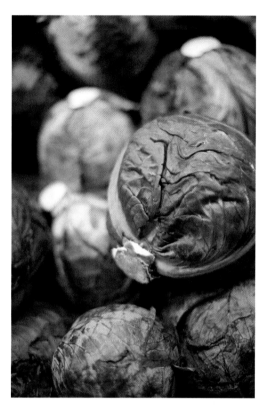

Carrots: One of my favorites! They're crunchy and sweet and packed with dietary fiber, vitamins A, C, and B6. Perfect for dipping.

Cauliflower: A good source of protein, thiamin, riboflavin, niacin and magnesium and phosphorus. It has a good amount of dietary fiber as well. Cauliflower is great roasted in the oven with garlic or steamed and mashed like a potato.

Celery: Grab a stalk and eat it raw. Celery is loaded with vitamin C, fiber, folate, potassium, and vitamins B1 and B6. And here's the great news: Celery is so low in calories and so high in fiber that you actually burn more calories eating and digesting it than the celery contains. It's great raw with a little cashew or almond butter; or try adding it to stir-fries for crunch. However you prepare it, celery should be in your life!

Chard: Vitamins C, E, and K, carotene, chlorophyll, and fiber—that's what chard is made of! It is also a good source of protein, calcium, selenium, zinc, niacin, and folate. Need any more reasons to put chard in your diet? It's one of the most popular vegetables in Mediterranean cooking, and it's great sautéed in a bit of olive oil with garlic and a squeeze of lemon juice or a sprinkling of red pepper flakes.

Corn: A good source of vitamins B1, B5 (pantothenic acid), C, and E, it also contains folate, magnesium, and phosphorus, and is a good source of complex carbohydrates, fiber, and essential fatty acids. Yellow corn is high in the carotenoid lutein, which can protect against heart disease and macular degeneration. Eat it boiled or grilled, on or off the cob, in salads, or added to soups and stews.

Cucumber: Because cucumber is very high in water, it is also very low in calories. But that doesn't mean it isn't nutritious. Cucumbers are a very good source of vitamins A and C and folate. The dark skin is also rich in fiber and minerals, including magnesium and potassium. Eat them raw in salads or by themselves, or make a cucumber salad with dill and rice vinegar—yum!

Eggplant: Rich in fiber and antioxidants, eggplant comes in many different colors, shapes, and sizes, all of which contain good amounts of B-complex vitamins, as well as minerals like manganese, copper, iron, and potassium. Eggplant is great sautéed, but it can soak up a lot of oil, so I'd recommend broiling or grilling it with a spritz of nonstick olive oil cooking spray.

Endive: There are actually several varieties of endive, including what most of us know as chicory and escarole. But you are probably most familiar with Belgian endive, which has lightly packed, flat leaves and looks sort of like a six-inch-long light green torpedo. It also is a good source of vitamin A and C. You can braise it or use it raw in salads—but be sure to wash it well, because those tightly packed leaves can be very sandy.

Garlic: So much can be said about this powerful little bulb! Maybe it doesn't really ward off evil spirits, but it has been shown to protect against some types of cancer and to lower cholesterol. Interestingly, studies indicate that chopping or crushing it and then allowing it to sit for fifteen minutes before cooking helps to release an enzyme that boosts its healthy compounds. If raw garlic is too strong for your taste, sautéing it makes its flavor a lot milder. Just don't burn it, because then it will turn bitter.

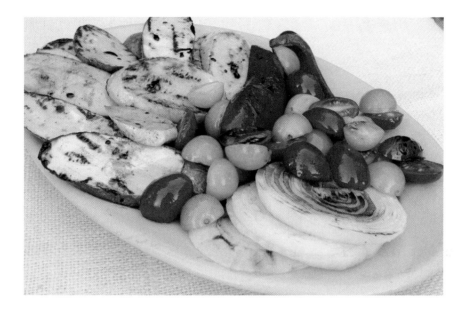

Green beans (string, snap, French): Protein and fiber are what green beans are known for. These beans are low in fat and high in complex carbohydrates. They are a good source of folate and molybdenum as well as iron, phosphorus, magnesium, manganese, and potassium. Try them cooked or raw. The benefits are endless.

Green peas contain a variety of antioxidants as well as vitamins C and E, zinc, and health-promoting omega-3 fatty acids. I love eating green peas right out of the shell, but I also love snow peas and sugar snap peas, both of which can be eaten pod and all, raw, cooked on their own, or in stir-fries—to name just a few of the ways to enjoy them.

Greens (collard, mustard, turnip, kale): Naturally high in fiber, greens help you fill up without filling out. And dark green leafy greens are loaded with beta-carotene, an antioxidant that helps to fight against cancer and heart disease. They are also great sources of vitamin C, folate, vitamin B6, manganese, and potassium. Greens are great raw in salads, steamed, or sautéed.

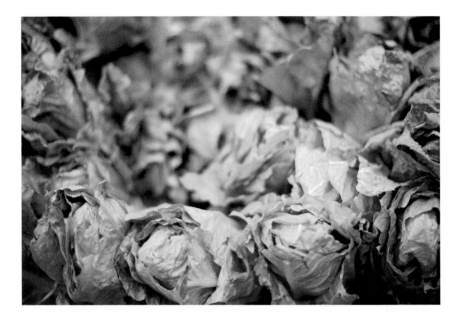

Hot peppers: If you like spicy, these are for you! The fire in hot peppers comes from capsaicin, which triggers the pain receptors in your mouth. Capsaicin has been shown to decrease blood cholesterol and triglyceride levels, boost immunity, and reduce the risk of stomach ulcers by killing bacteria in the stomach that can lead to ulcers. Not all hot peppers are created equal, and their heat is measured on what is called the Scoville scale from hottest to mildest. To see the ratings, go online to scovillescaleforpeppers.com. To make your dish milder, seed and rinse the peppers before using them (just remember to wash your hands after you handle them to avoid inadvertently rubbing your eyes—that smarts!), and use fewer, to accommodate your tolerance for spice.

Leeks: One of my favorites! Leeks provide fiber, folate, vitamins C and B6, and important minerals like manganese and iron. Anything that you do with onions or garlic, you can also do with leeks.

Lettuce (all types): The varieties are endless! Lettuce is mostly made of water, but some varieties offer more nutrients than others, including beta-carotene, folate, vitamin C, and potassium. The rock stars are radicchio, arugula, endive, chicory, and escarole, but all lettuce is also a great source of fiber. Grab a mix and make a salad!

Mushrooms: I've included mushrooms among the vegetables, but actually they're a type of fungus (sorry)! They're high in water and fiber, which means they're low in calories, and they have numerous health benefits, including potassium, riboflavin, selenium, and niacin. Mushrooms come in so many varieties, from meaty portobellos to pungent crimini, tiny mild enoki, and regular white, that there must be a mushroom for every taste and every occasion. Have them raw in salads, use them in vegetarian stews, add them to stir-fries, or combine them with other vegetables or legumes—to name just a few of the many ways to incorporate mushrooms into your diet.

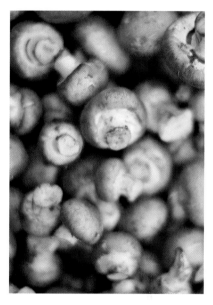

Okra: Although it's best known in the South for its use in gumbo, anybody anywhere can benefit from okra. It is loaded with vitamins B6 and C as well as fiber, calcium, and folate. It is known to be effective for the prevention of neural tube defects in developing fetuses. Okra is great steamed or sautéed; combined with tomatoes, a little thyme, and a bay leaf, it makes a great vegetarian stew.

Onions, scallions, and shallots: Onions and their cousins provide vitamins B6 and C, chromium, biotin, and fiber. They also contain folate, provide vitamins B1 and K, and are believed to protect against heart disease, lower inflammation at the cellular level, and reduce the risk of prostate cancer. Not to mention that they are delicious cooked or raw, in almost any meal, and come in many varieties from sweet to pungent.

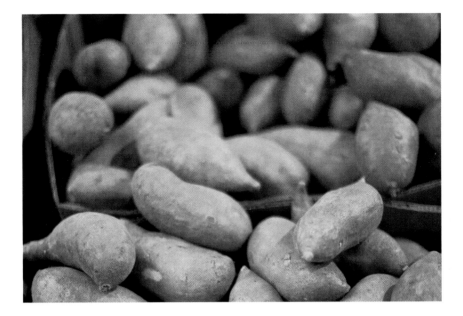

Potatoes, sweet: I love all kinds of potatoes, and I believe they've gotten a bad rap by being called "fattening." Sweet potatoes in particular have significant health benefits, with possibly more bioavailable (meaning that our bodies are able to use it) beta-carotene than any other vegetable. Despite the fact that they are, in fact, a starchy vegetable, recent studies have shown that they actually help to control blood sugar rather than raising it.

Potatoes, white: White potatoes aren't bad either. They are a good source of vitamin B6, vitamin C, copper, potassium, manganese, and fiber. In fact, a baked potato has more potassium than any other vegetable and more than a banana. And they also have significant antioxidant properties. In addition, British scientists at the Institute of Food Research have recently identified blood-pressure-lowering compounds called kukoamines in potatoes. One medium baked potato has only about 150 calories. It's the way we cook potatoes (such as deep-frying) and the stuff we love to put on them (butter and sour cream) that can make what is essentially a healthy food unhealthy.

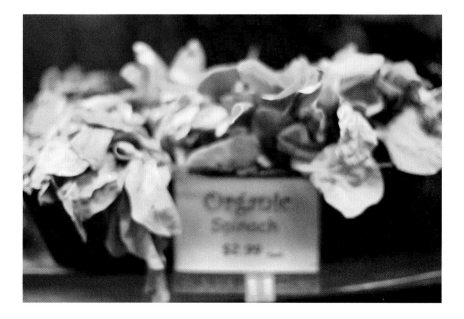

Radishes: Some say their flavor takes a little getting used to, but radishes are high in vitamin C, are a good source of calcium, and contain compounds that have been shown to protect against colon cancer. Eat one raw, like an apple, or add them to salads for extra zing.

Spinach contains more nutrients than almost any other vegetable. It is a major source of vitamins C and K, cancer-fighting carotenes, and folate, and also contains significant amounts of manganese, iron, magnesium, and vitamins B2, B1, B6, and E. Just so you know, the iron content of spinach is twice that of other greens (so Popeye was right!) and it is one of the most alkaline foods you can find, meaning that it helps to regulate the body's pH balance. Spinach is great for promoting eye health by preventing macular degeneration and cataracts. Eat it raw in salads, steamed, or sautéed—just be sure to eat it often!

Sprouts (all types) are loaded with antioxidants, protein, chlorophyll, vitamins, minerals, and amino acids. Ever heard of wheatgrass? The juice is considered to be the closest substance to hemoglobin and is therefore an amazing blood purifier and liver detoxifier. Sprouts come in many varieties and flavors and are great in salads, so be adventurous.

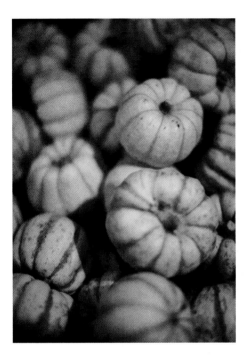

Squash comes in many shapes and colors and is known for its fiber content as well as for containing good amounts of vitamin C, beta-carotene, and folate. It is credited with helping to prevent many cancers and heart disease, as well as the inflammation associated with arthritis and asthma. Baked, sautéed, steamed, or stir-fried, squash is fabulous.

Tomato: See Fruits (that's right: A tomato is a fruit).

Turnips: Similar to potatoes in texture, turnips have a slightly bitter flavor. They contain vitamin C and many B vitamins, including riboflavin, thiamin, niacin, folate, and pantothenic acid. Turnips are also great sources of fiber and pair well with naturally sweet meats like pork. Try them mashed instead of potatoes!

Zucchini: Though it's actually a summer squash, we've come to think of zucchini as a vegetable in a category all its own. It's an important source of potassium, which helps to lower blood pressure; B vitamins like thiamin, pyridoxine, and riboflavin; and minerals such as iron, manganese, phosphorus, and zinc. Have it grilled, steamed, or sautéed with almost any meal.

Fruits

Apples contain pectin, a fat-soluble fiber that, in combination with other apple phytonutrients, has been shown to lower blood fat. They also contain good amounts of vitamin C, potassium, and health-promoting polyphenols—which have been shown to help control blood sugar—and have many other health benefits as well. So an apple a day may really help keep the doctor away. They come in so many varieties that there's surely one to suit your taste. And they give you a lot of "chew" and satisfaction for your calorie buck.

Apricots: These are yet another orange-colored food that's high in beta-carotene and vitamin A. Researchers involved in the Nurses' Health Study, one of the longest-running and most comprehensive studies of women's health, found that those with the highest intake of vitamin A reduced their risk of developing cataracts by 40 percent. And one apricot has only 17 calories! When they're in season (approximately May through August) enjoy one freshly picked or with half a cup of 2 percent cottage cheese.

Avocado: They're one of the best sources of potassium and contain good amounts of vitamins B and E. While they are very high in fat, more than half their total fat is in the form of monounsaturated oleic acid, which has been shown to lower the risk for heart disease. In addition, research has shown that, when eaten in combination, avocado can increase the absorption of carotenoids (which are powerful antioxidants) from other foods—and the

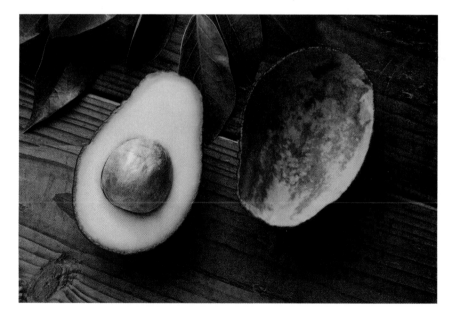

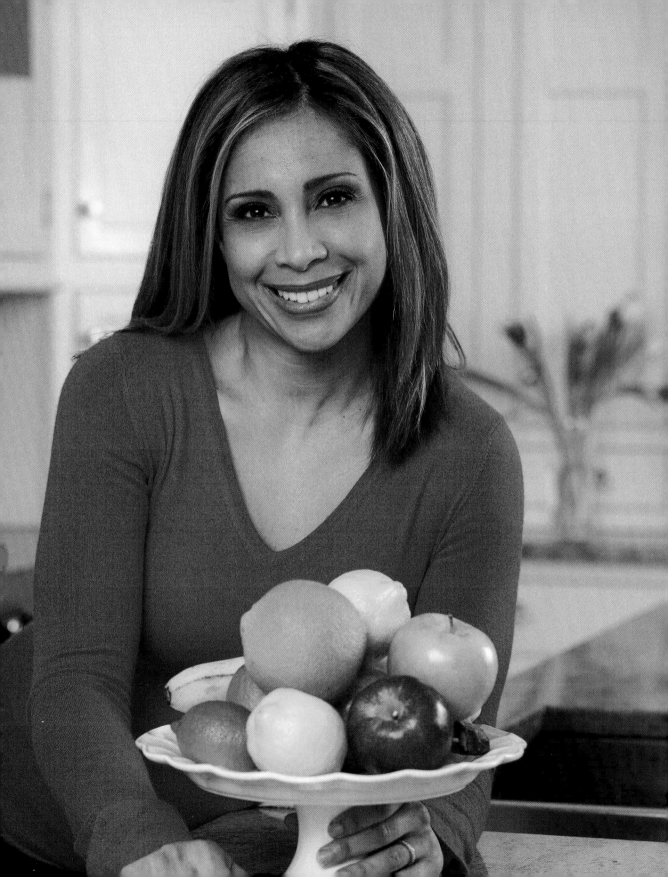

avocado itself contains a wide variety of carotenoids. Add them to salads or mash a ripe avocado with tomato, onion, and cilantro to make a delicious guacamole. Just don't overdo—healthy or not, fat is high in calories.

Bananas: Extremely high in potassium, bananas also contain vitamins C and B6 as well as loads of fiber, magnesium, carbohydrates, riboflavin, and biotin. The riper the banana the sweeter it is, because the starch is turning to sugar. Bananas, while they're certainly healthy, are also high on the glycemic index.

Blackberries: In addition to vitamins C and E, blackberries are a super source of polyphenols and anthocyanins, two types of antioxidant that can help to protect against many types of chronic diseases. And of course, they are delicious. Eat them alone or in combination with other health-promoting berries.

Blueberries have one of the highest antioxidant capacities of all fruits and vegetables. In addition, they are a great source of fiber, vitamin C, manganese, and riboflavin. And at least one recent study has shown that they may help to improve memory in older adults and so might help to postpone the onset of cognitive problems related to aging. Although they are not usually considered "low" on the glycemic index, recent studies have shown that people already diagnosed with Type 2 diabetes who eat blueberries along with other low-glycemic fruits for a period of three months showed a significant increase in their ability to control blood sugar. So go ahead and eat your blueberries—they're good for you.

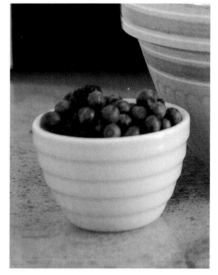

Cantaloupe and honeydew melon: They're fat-free, juicy, sweet, and good sources of potassium and vitamin C. Have them for breakfast, a snack, or even dessert.

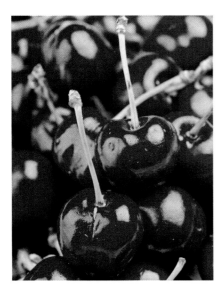

Cherries: Gorgeous! Anthocyanins, which give cherries their color, are natural pain relievers and anti-inflammatories. They also contain melatonin, which helps to regulate sleep cycles; are rich in fiber and vitamin C; and contain iron, copper, manganese, potassium, and zinc. Tart cherries in particular are rich in lutein, zeaxanthin, and beta-carotene, antioxidants that help fight aging, reduce the risk of heart disease, and may have anticancer properties. Eat them alone or with other fruits for breakfast, a snack, or dessert.

Cranberries: Can you say vitamin C! Cranberries are also packed with soluble and insoluble fiber, as well as manganese and copper. And like cherries, blueberries, and other dark red or purple fruits, they are a rich source of the antioxidant pigment anthocyanin. Drinking cranberry juice helps to prevent and treat urinary tract infections, and a compound found in cranberries also blocks plaque formation on teeth. Try naturally sweetened cranberries in salads or unsweetened applesauce.

Grapes: Another all-star among fruits, grapes have endless benefits. Packed with phytonutrients, vitamins, and minerals, they have powerful antioxidant properties and have been shown to protect against cancer, heart disease, degenerative nerve disease, Alzheimer's disease, and viral/fungal infections. There are many varieties; try them all.

Kiwi: These have a beautiful bright green color and are a very good source of vitamins C, A, E, and K. Kiwis also contain flavonoid antioxidants including beta-carotene, lutein, and xanthin.

They are a rich source of soluble dietary fiber and omega-3 fatty acids. Peel one and try it sliced with Greek yogurt, in a fruit salad, or on its own.

Mangoes: I love mangoes! They are rich in dietary fiber, vitamin A, minerals, and beta-carotene. New research has shown mangoes to be helpful in protecting against leukemia as well as colon, breast, and prostate cancers.

Orange: Like other citrus fruits, oranges are an excellent source of vitamin C, as well as fiber and vitamin A. The antioxidants in oranges have also been found to help in preventing many cancers as well as chronic diseases like arthritis. To get the greatest effect from all these nutrients as well as the fiber, eat an orange rather than drinking its juice.

Peaches: The ancient Chinese considered the peach a symbol of longevity, and it turns out they were probably right. Peaches are good sources of potassium, beta-carotene, and vitamin C. They

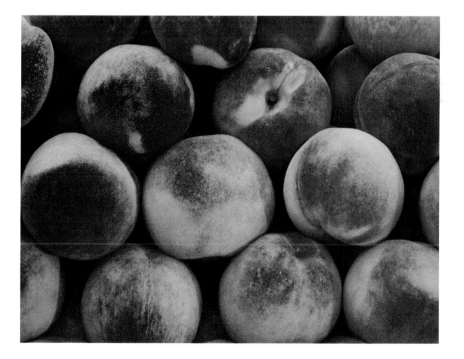

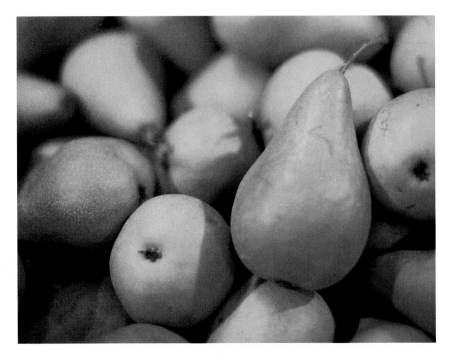

also contain lycopene and lutein, which studies have found to protect against macular degeneration, heart disease, and cancer. And besides, what could be better than a ripe, juicy peach on a hot summer day!

Pears: High in fiber, antioxidants, minerals, and vitamins, pears promote colon and heart health and may offer protection against colon cancer. Pears come in many varieties; try a few and find your favorite.

Pineapple: Known for containing bromelain, an enzyme that digests food by breaking down protein, pineapple has also been shown to have anti-inflammatory, anticlotting, and anticancer properties. And nothing is more delicious than a ripe, juicy pineapple.

Plums: There are so many kinds with so many flavors that I almost feel they're different kinds of fruit. They come in various colors, but the easiest to find are the red and purple varieties. Plums

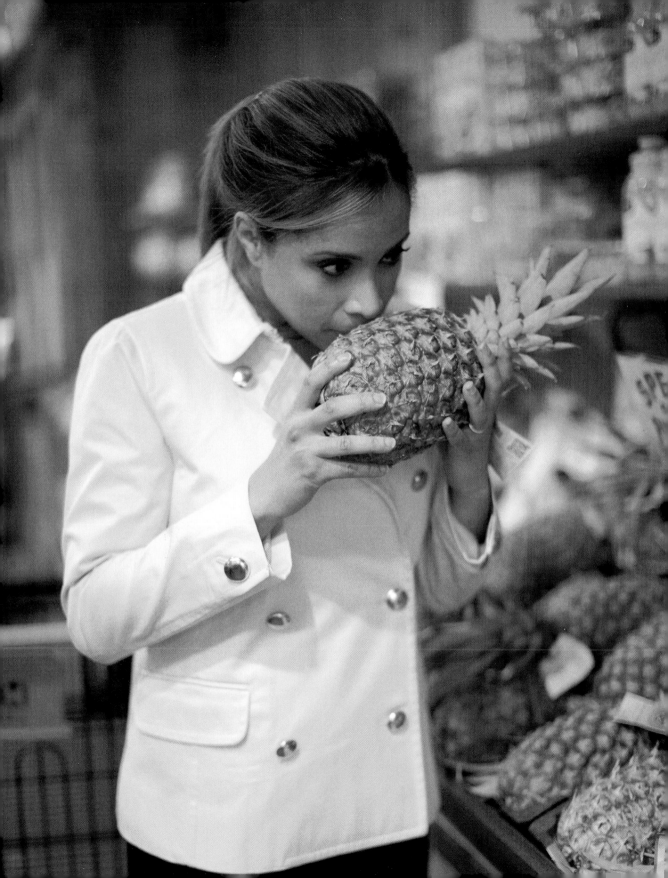

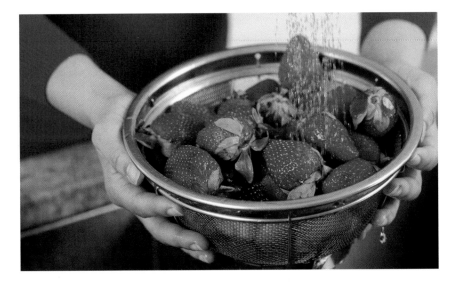

increase the body's ability to absorb iron and are a very good source of vitamin C. Have a plum with some Greek yogurt, or stew them with other fruits to make a compote.

Raspberries: Along with other dark red or purple berries, raspberries are rich in antioxidants that reduce inflammation, fight aging, and offer protection against cancer. They are also an excellent source of vitamins C, A, and E. Eat them as a snack, in fruit salads, or with yogurt.

Strawberries: These luscious berries contain vitamins A, C, E, and B-complex as well as potassium, manganese, fluorine, copper, iron, and iodine. They are also low cal and low on the glycemic index, so enjoy them at any time of the day.

Tomatoes: Considered a superfood because of their great antioxidant properties, tomatoes have been shown to protect against colon, prostate, breast, endometrial, lung, skin, and pancreatic cancer. Cooking tomatoes actually makes more of their antioxidants available for use in your body, so stew them and use them in sauces. Canned plum tomatoes are a great alternative when good tomatoes are hard to find, but don't forget to enjoy a delicious, ripe local tomato at the height of the summer season.

Watermelon has a lot of sugar (which is why it's so sweet) but also a lot of—well—water, which means that its glycemic load is relatively low, and it's also very low in calories. Watermelon contains vitamins C and A as well as potassium and magnesium. So if you want a sweet treat at the end of your meal, have a piece of watermelon. Or try it in a salad with sweet red onion and fresh mint.

Legumes

Defined as plants that bear edible seeds in pods, legumes actually include peas and green beans, which I've included in the vegetable category because that's what most of us consider them. When we think of legumes, we think mostly of the beans we generally buy dried or canned, already out of their pods. Soybeans, lentils, and peanuts are also legumes.

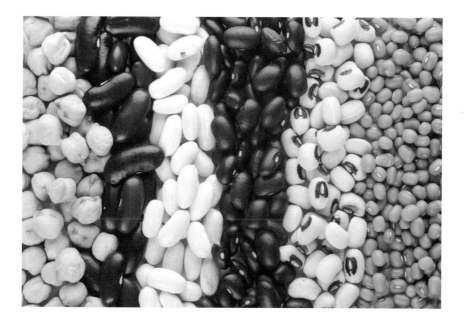

These are an important source of protein and fiber and are also high in B vitamins, folic acid, iron, calcium, potassium, and magnesium. They have been shown to help lower cholesterol and blood pressure, regulate blood sugar, and protect against some types of cancer.

While the protein in legumes (except for soybeans) is not "complete" because it doesn't provide all the essential amino acids found only in animal sources, legumes, unlike most animal proteins, contain very little fat, and the fat they do contain is not saturated.

While the variety is huge, the legumes we encounter most often include black beans (used copiously in Mexican food), cannellini, chickpeas (aka garbanzos), fava beans, great northern, kidney, lima, navy, and pinto. Be adventurous; try them all, in salads, stews, or as a side dish.

Grains

Amaranth: An ancient food of the Aztecs, amaranth is a tiny yellow grain with a sweet peppery taste that goes well with many vegetables including broccoli, carrots, onions, and red peppers. It is gluten-free and one of only two grains that provide complete protein—quinoa is the other (see below). It also contains linoleic acid and lysine, two essential fatty acids that we must get from food sources. In addition, amaranth is an excellent source of fiber and a great source of iron, magnesium, and calcium. It can help prevent anemia and osteoporosis and has been linked to reducing the risks of heart disease, cancers, and digestive-tract conditions. Look for it in your local health food store, boil some up, and eat it as a hot cereal, like pilaf, or use it to make a tabouli salad.

Barley: The US Department of Agriculture reports that diets high in barley were found to lower total cholesterol levels. It has also been found to help reduce high blood pressure in men. Originally from Ethiopia and Southeast Asia, barley has been around for more than ten thousand years. It is packed with dietary fiber and selenium (an antioxidant), and is also a good source of phosphorus, copper, and manganese. Barley is great in soups and stews; or you can eat it instead of pasta.

Cornmeal: This is a whole grain made from ground corn. It contains many nutrients including niacin, thiamine, riboflavin, pantothenic acid, folate, and vitamins B6, E, and K, as well as valuable minerals such as iron, magnesium, phosphorus, potassium, zinc, copper, manganese, and selenium. Be sure that if you buy cornmeal, it actually is whole grain; otherwise it will have lost much of its nutritional value.

Oatmeal (steel cut): Steel-cut oats are different from traditional rolled oats. Steel-cut oats are just that—oat kernels that have been cut into two or three pieces with steel blades. Rolled oats are

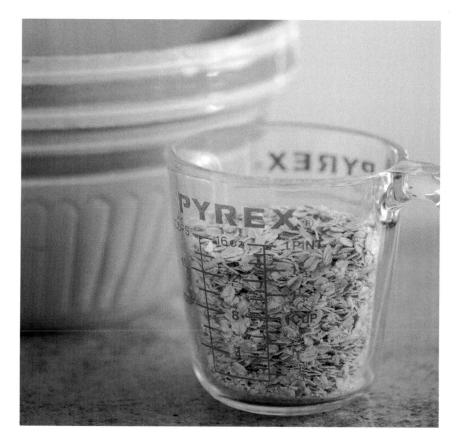

rolled flat with most of the bran removed to make them quicker to cook, but they also have much less fiber than steel-cut oats. Oats have been shown to help control blood sugar and lower cholesterol, which makes steel-cut oatmeal a good choice for breakfast.

Quinoa (pronounced KEEN-wah): Like amaranth, quinoa is a source of complete protein. It is also a good source of riboflavin (vitamin B2), which has been shown to reduce the frequency of migraine headaches, and magnesium, which helps to reduce blood pressure and increase cardiovascular health. Eat it instead of oatmeal for breakfast, mix it into salads, or serve it as a pilaf-like side dish.

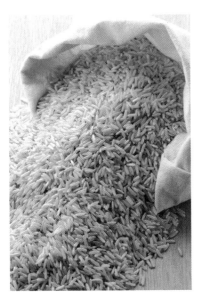

Rice (brown): Much less processed than white rice, brown rice has only the outer hull removed, preserving the bran and most of the germ—along with most of its nutrients. It is high in fiber, an excellent source of manganese, and a good source of selenium and magnesium. It has a great chewy texture and a nutty flavor. Serve it whenever you would otherwise use white rice.

Rye/pumpernickel: Rye is a grain generally used to make bread. Pumpernickel bread is a dark, somewhat sour bread made from whole coarsely ground rye. Rye contain loads of fiber, antioxidants including vitamin E and selenium, iron, magnesium, zinc, and B vitamins. Just be sure that the bread you buy is made from whole rye and not mixed with refined white flour, as many commercial products are.

Spelt: One of my favorites! A cousin of wheat but with more protein and minerals, spelt has a sweet, nutty flavor. It is packed with niacin (vitamin B3), which is needed for proper circulation and helps to reduce cholesterol levels in the blood. Since it has a high water solubility, spelt is said to be easier to digest for those with a wheat intolerance. Spelt makes amazing bread.

Whole wheat: Simply put, this is wheat in its unrefined state, which means that it retains virtually all of its nutritional benefits. It is packed with fiber, has good amounts of vitamins E, B6, and K, and also contains magnesium, iron, calcium, potassium, and zinc. Like other whole grain foods, whole wheat helps to reduce the risk of cancer and cardiovascular disease. Choose whole wheat pastas and breads, and read the labels carefully to be sure that what you're buying really is 100 percent whole wheat.

Wild rice: Guess what—wild rice isn't actually a member of the rice family, although it is a grain-producing grass. It's full of antioxidants and has twice as much protein as brown rice. It also contains important vitamins and minerals including folate, niacin, phosphorus, and zinc. Use it whenever you would otherwise serve brown rice.

As you will have noticed, the legumes and some of the grains discussed above contain significant amounts of protein. Following are the Quick & Clean animal foods that we generally think of when we are thinking about protein.

Fish

All of the fish listed here are rich in essential omega-3 fatty acids as well as other heart-healthy vitamins and minerals. Fish is low in fat and calories, and should be part of any healthy diet. The only caveat is that some fish—tuna in particular—may contain mercury and should, therefore, be eaten sparingly, particular by women who are pregnant or planning to become pregnant. If you're in doubt, check with your health care provider.

Cod: One of my favorites! This is a mild-flavored white, cold-water fish that's easily available all year round.

Halibut: A firm, white-meat fish with a delicate sweet flavor, halibut is a favorite among those who think they really don't like fish. Try it; you'll probably like it!

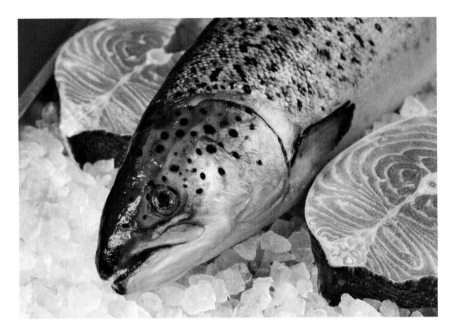

Salmon: A rock star among fish! Wild salmon is better than farmed, and wild Alaskan salmon is the best-of-the-best. When you're eating wild Alaskan salmon, you don't have to worry about mercury.

Sardines: In addition to their other health benefits, these small, saltwater, soft-boned fish from the Mediterranean are a great source of tryptophan, a precursor to the production of the neurotransmitter serotonin that provides a sense of well-being and promotes sound sleep. Try them in a salad instead of tuna.

Scallops: I love both the tiny bay scallops and the larger sea scallops. They are a very good source of vitamin B12 and omega-3 fatty acids, and a good source of magnesium, potassium, and other nutrients that supply significant cardiovascular benefits.

Shrimp are so quick and easy to cook, and go well with so many other ingredients, that you will find several shrimp recipes in this book. They are a low-fat, low-calorie protein and contain a good amount of vitamin B12 and omega-3 fatty acids, both of which are known to protect against heart disease and help to lower blood sugar levels.

Meat

Beef can be extremely high in unhealthy saturated fat, and it can also be full of harmful pesticides and hormones. I do eat beef, but only the leanest cuts from organic, grass-fed cattle, which I appreciate can be expensive. The leanest cuts are "round," which is taken from the back leg bone; flank steak, which comes from the abdominal muscles; and tenderloin, which comes from the tenderloin muscle. Tenderloin, as the name implies, is extremely tender and good for grilling. Both the round and the flank are much less tender and, therefore, require relatively long cooking. You'll find a recipe for flank steak in chapter 14.

Buffalo meat: Lower in fat than most cuts of beef, buffalo is rich in vitamins and minerals, tends to have more iron than beef, and can be prepared in the same ways as its beef cousin.

Calf's liver: Liver can be a tough sell, so hear the facts. It's packed with vitamins A, Bs (riboflavin), and D, and is loaded with iron and copper. It's also low in fat and calories. Try it grilled with onions. Maybe the onions will do it for you.

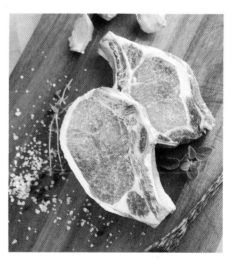

Nitrite-free turkey bacon is the only exception to the Quick & Clean embargo on cured meats (see chapter 6).

Pork: A lean, white meat, pork is high in thiamin and lower in salt than other meats. It's also a great source of iron and is rich in vitamin B12 and zinc. It's sweet tasting and can be prepared in a variety of ways. Pork tenderloin is great for grilling, and you'll find a Quick & Clean pork chop recipe in chapter 14.

Poultry (white-meat chicken, turkey, and Cornish hen): A low-fat alternative to beef, white-meat poultry is a generous source of B vitamins and other nutrients. There are many types of poultry with different flavors. It is easy to prepare and very versatile. Try some of the recipes in chapter 14 or do it "your way."

Fats

Canola oil: Among the healthiest of cooking oils, canola oil has less saturated fat than any other oil commonly consumed in the United States, including olive oil. In fact, there is enough evidence for the heart-healthy benefits of this oil that the Food and Drug Administration allows manufacturers to make a qualified health claim on their label. And because it has a much lighter flavor than olive oil, it is the better choice for cooking when you don't want the flavor of the oil to interfere with the flavor of the food.

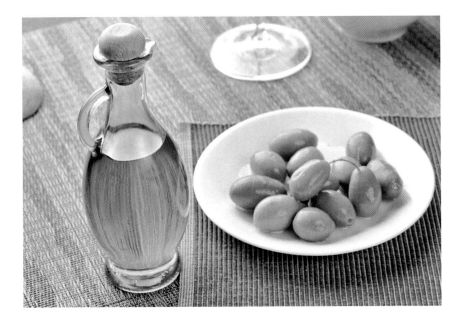

Extra-virgin olive oil: Olive oil is a monounsaturated fat that has been shown to reduce blood pressure, inhibit some cancers, and stave off heart disease by controlling bad (LDL) cholesterol levels while raising good ones (HDL). "Extra virgin" is the highest quality and purest of the many types of olive oil on the market. In addition to using it in salad dressings and for cooking, try dipping whole grain bread into it instead of butter—the way the Italians do!

Flaxseed oil: Recent studies are indicating that flaxseed oil has significant health benefits, as it is a plant source for omega-3 fatty acids, which are generally found mostly in fish. It also contains estrogen-like compounds called lignans that studies have shown to be protective against breast cancer. It's not good for cooking because heating it can destroy its health benefits, but it's great in salad dressings, and I also use it to make my Mixed Berry and Flaxseed Oil Super Smoothie (chapter 14).

Safflower oil: Often confused with sunflower oil, safflower oil has a light, delicate flavor; is low in saturated fat; and is high in both omega-6 fatty acids, which may help to burn fat, and vitamin E. Use it for cooking or in salad dressings.

Dairy

Cheese: There are so many different kinds of cheese that it would be impossible to even begin to talk about them individually. Like other dairy products, cheese is a good source of protein and is high in calcium, which is good for bone health. But cheese can also be high in fat, so you should eat it sparingly. In general, hard cheeses are lower in fat than soft ones. As you can imagine, cheeses labeled "triple crème" are extremely high in fat, while string cheese, for example, has a relatively low fat content. So do your homework, compare flavors and fat, and enjoy cheese as a snack, with fruit, or as a garnish—just don't overindulge.

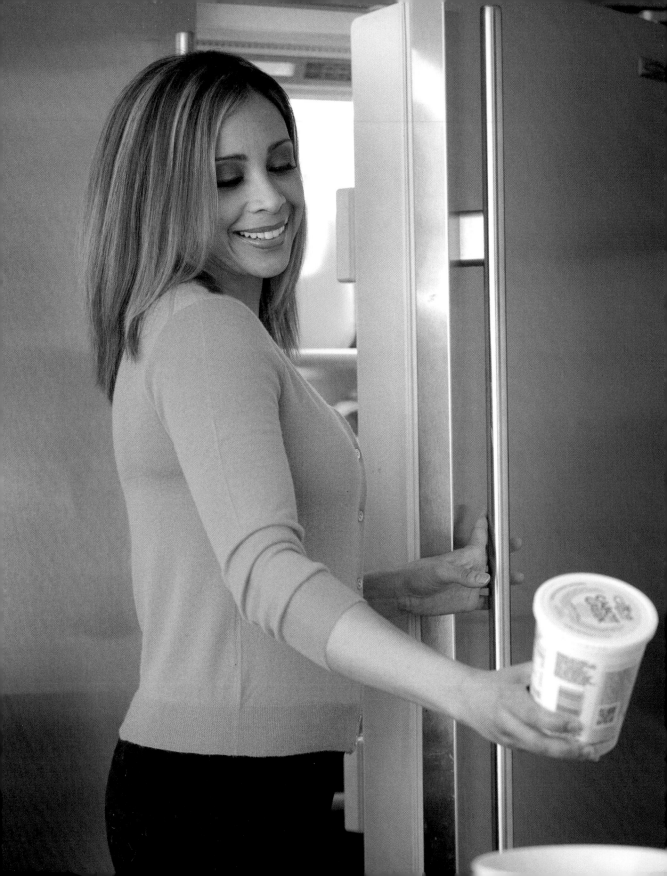

Eggs: I learned to love them. Eggs contain super high quality protein and are very clean. They're packed with vitamins and minerals and keep you full for a long time. If cholesterol is a problem for you, just stay away from the yolks.

Greek yogurt: The new star among health-conscious foodies, Greek yogurt has more protein and less sugar than regular yogurt. It's also richer and creamier because the water and whey have been strained out, but you should know it also has a slightly bitter taste that may take some getting used to. Look for low-fat varieties (I use 2 percent fat and also nonfat), and try it with fruit.

Kefir: A fermented milk drink, kefir is a probiotic known to restore the balance of intestinal flora for digestive health. It is also a source of complete protein and is rich in vitamins and minerals. Look for it in a variety of flavors near the yogurt in your supermarket.

Milk: Most of us need milk sometimes, but we certainly don't need all the fat in whole milk. I use skim milk as well as 1 and 2 percent milk. My advice is to go as low fat as you can. Or try light soy milk.

Sweeteners

Agave: The natural sweetener agave is quickly becoming a favorite in the kitchen. Once associated with making tequila, it is now becoming an alternative to table sugar. Agave comes from the leaves of the Agave americana plant. The nectar is expressed from the leaves, then filtered and heated. Because it is composed mainly of fructose and glucose, it has a lower glycemic index than sucrose (table sugar). It comes in light (or golden) and dark (or amber) varieties. The light kind is heated to lower temperatures in processing and tastes milder. The dark, which is heated to higher temperatures, tastes more like molasses or maple syrup. Agave dissolves easily and can be used as a sweetener in any dish, sauce, dressing, or dessert. A little goes a long way.

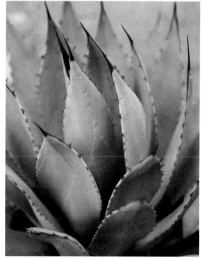

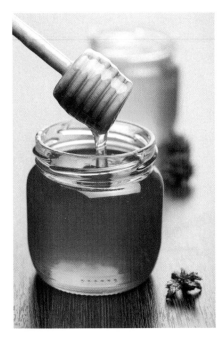

Raw honey: Dr. Oz calls this "liquid gold" because of its healing properties. Raw honey hasn't been filtered, strained, or heated, so it retains all its nutrients. It's rich in vitamins B1, B2, B3, B5, and B6 as well as vitamin C; it contains minerals including magnesium, potassium, calcium, sodium, sulfur, and phosphate. It is known to have antibacterial and antifungal properties and makes a great alternative to Neosporin (yep!). Because of its immune-boosting, antiviral properties, raw honey has been used in the treatment of ulcers, diarrhea, bronchitis, and gastrointestinal problems. A sweetener with health benefits—how sweet is that! If you can buy it organic, go for it.

Stevia: A zero-calorie sugar substitute that comes from the stevia plant, this sweetener is twenty-five to thirty times sweeter than sugar in addition to being far healthier. Stevia comes in both granule and liquid form and in a variety of flavors. It has a zero glycemic index and is recommended for diabetics. It can be added to all types of foods and is particularly great for sweetening desserts.

Truvia is a natural, stevia-based sugar substitute that comes in powder form and can be used in the same way as table sugar. If you have a sweet tooth, this is a good option for any stage of the Quick & Clean Diet.

Xylitol: A sugar alcohol sweetener commonly used as a sugar substitute, xylitol occurs naturally in the fibers of many fruits and vegetables and can be extracted from various berries, oats, and mushrooms. Xylitol is commonly found in breath mints and chewing gum and is considered safe for diabetics because it has almost no effect on insulin levels and is not easily converted to fat. Some studies have shown that xylitol may even help improve bone density and could be a potential treatment for osteoporosis.

There are many of claims of health benefits for xylitol, but there are some warnings too. One in particular that you need to know about is that in excess xylitol, like many sugar alcohols, can have a laxative effect, causing temporary gastrointestinal effects like bloating, flatulence, and diarrhea. So if you are interested in using xylitol as a sugar substitute, don't go crazy. It can be purchased in a powder form—much like a bag of sugar—from health food stores.

We just took a look at foods to love, and in the next chapter we'll explore ways to spice up your dishes. The best part of what I call your Q & C pantry partners is that they're packed with flavor and very few calories!

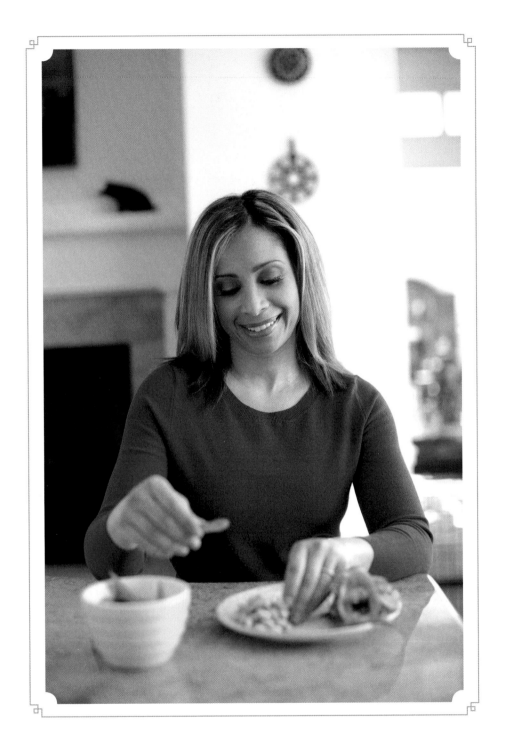

Five

Your Quick & Clean Pantry Partners

When you think of losing weight, I bet you think, *To shed pounds, I have to lose my taste buds.* No way! Healthy food does not lack flavor. As I've said from the beginning, I love to eat, and I want my food to be intensely flavorful. I would never stand for bland, boring food, and neither should you! When you're trying to make a big change in your eating habits is exactly the time when you should *not* feel deprived.

The herbs, spices, and other flavor enhancers I'll be talking about in this chapter can be used freely in every stage of the Quick & Clean Diet and will ensure that your taste buds remain happy as your waist size goes down. Some of them may be new to you, so I urge you to be open-minded and adventurous. You are embarking on a big change, so why not pick up a few new favorites along the way! The idea is to gain nutrition and lose fat, all while enjoying the process.

Fresh Herbs

A must-have! Fresh herbs can be found in almost any supermarket, and you can even grow them in your backyard or right on your kitchen windowsill. There's nothing like the aroma that arises when you pick a sprig of thyme or a few fresh basil leaves. Their flavors can be subtle or bold, and you can use as much or as little as you like. Herbs are great for infusing flavor into meats, fish, vegetables, salads, grains, and even desserts.

Here are a few you may already be familiar with and that you certainly should try.

Basil: The aroma is legendary. There's nothing more fresh and fragrant than a summer tomato and basil salad with a hint of pepper

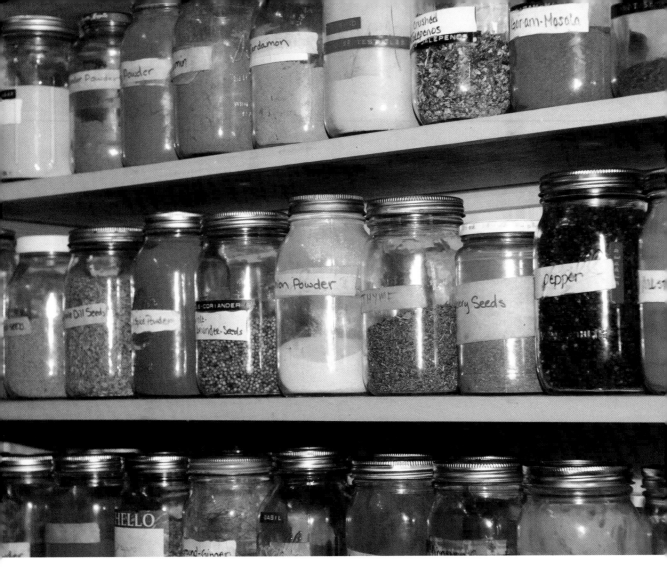

and olive oil! Basil is used for making pesto, as well as many other sauces. The leaves are great fresh-picked in sandwiches, soups, and salads. I love to include basil in my salad dressings and even add it to fruit desserts. In terms of health benefits, basil contains flavonoid and carotenoid antioxidants and antibacterial properties associated with its volatile oils. It is a good source of magnesium, potassium, and vitamin C, and a very good source of iron and calcium.

Chives are the Chihuahuas of the onion family—they're small but feisty. Chop them fine and use them as a garnish for soups, in omelets, with fish, with vegetables, and in dips. Chives help lower blood pressure, are rich in vitamins A and C, and contain trace amounts of sulfur and iron. Sprinkle them on salads or over fish.

Cilantro: The leafy portion of the coriander seed, cilantro is used in some Latin American countries as a remedy for an upset stomach. It can look a lot like flat-leaf parsley, but its leaves are much smaller and its flavor is much more pungent. A staple of Mexican and Indian cooking, it's becoming ever more popular as an herb in the United States. So yes, use it in homemade salsa and guacamole, but also try it with chicken, in turkey burgers, with fish, and with vegetables. It is a good source of potassium, calcium, manganese, iron, and magnesium as well as folate, riboflavin, niacin, vitamin A, vitamin C, and beta-carotene.

Cilantro is admittedly not to everyone's taste. I've found that you either love it or loathe it. If you love it, use it liberally; if not, try parsley instead.

Dill: A wispy, delicate herb that adds a great little twist to many dishes. It's great in omelets and sprinkled on top of fish; or try it in sauces or light soups. Dill is rich in antioxidants and many vitamins including folate, riboflavin, niacin, vitamin A, and vitamin C.

Mint: This sassy herb is popular in many Mediterranean dishes, and mint is often served with lamb as well as in salads. Use it to add zing to grain and vegetable dishes. Mint comes in many, many varieties, so try a few to see which ones you like best. It's also rich in antioxidants and contains menthol, a natural pain reliever.

Oregano: Of Mediterranean origin, the word oregano derives from the Greek and means "joy of the mountains." With its potent aroma and taste, it is great sprinkled on just about anything. We know it as a key ingredient in tomato sauce, but oregano is also

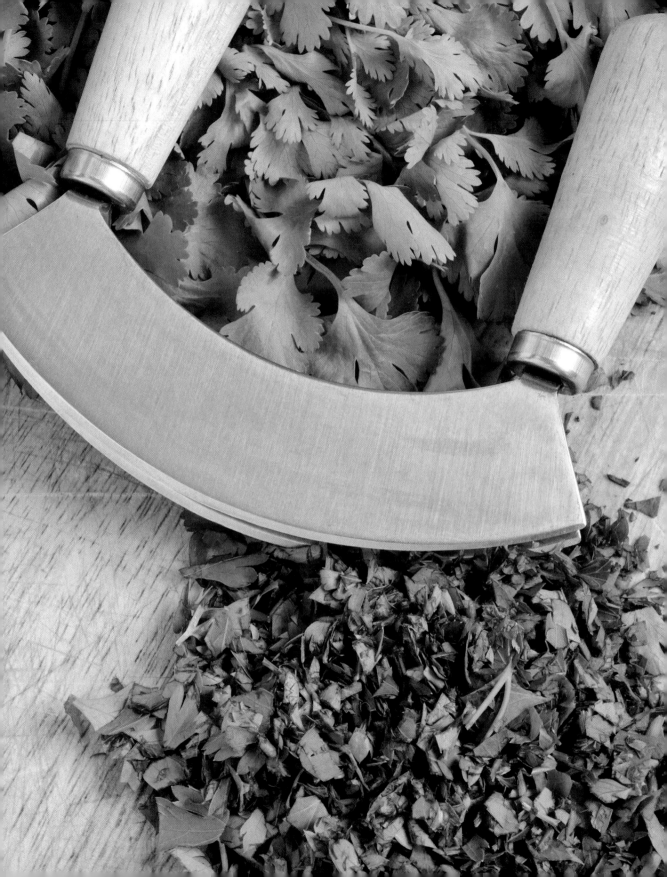

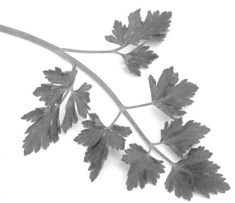

wonderful with poultry, seafood, vegetables, and in salads. One warning: If you use too much in a dish, it can leave a slightly bitter aftertaste. A little is magic. As far as your health goes, oregano contains an essential oil called thymol that is known to have antibacterial and antifungal properties. It's also high in vitamin C and contains effective antioxidants.

Parsley: I want to say this herb can be used in just about everything! You've probably seen both the curly and flat varieties. The flat, or Italian, parsley is what I use in cooking. I think of the curly variety as more of a garnish to make the platter pretty. It works wonders chopped with garlic on top of meats, poultry, fish, vegetables, and in soups. It's great in a salad dressing. It's brilliant with lemon. And when it comes to health, parsley is rich in antioxidants, vitamins, minerals, and dietary fiber. It's definitely an herb that should be on your weekly shopping list!

Rosemary: A very aromatic herb with a woody fragrance whose name means "dew of the sea" in Latin. Extremely versatile, it can be used in many dishes, including soups, vegetables, meats, poultry (try putting a sprig or two in the cavity of a chicken before roasting), salads, stuffings, and even desserts. It is rich in folate and other B vitamins and is a good source of iron and calcium.

On a personal note . . .

I prefer using fresh herbs whenever possible because their flavor is—well—fresher, and because when they're dried they lose much of the vitamin and mineral content. But if you can't find fresh, by all means use dried. They work just fine in most dishes. Remember, the flavor will be different and also more concentrated, so you'll need less.

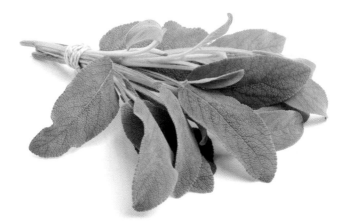

Sage: With its long, narrow, slightly fuzzy, grayish green leaf and musky flavor, sage is a staple in stuffings, particularly around Thanksgiving. But it also is great with pork, pasta, and all kinds of poultry. Sage is a good source of B-complex vitamins such as folate, as well as vitamin A and beta-carotene.

Tarragon is especially popular in France, but we Americans love it too! It's bittersweet, with a licorice-like fragrance that pairs wonderfully with chicken, pork, fish, and many vegetables. It also works well with eggs and in hearty soups. Tarragon is great in a mustard or citrus sauce or chopped in a salad dressing. Rich in antioxidants, it's considered an excellent source of minerals, including calcium, manganese, iron, magnesium, copper, potassium, and zinc.

Thyme: One of my very favorites! Thyme comes in many varieties, including French thyme, English thyme, golden lemon, silver lemon, orange, lime, and more. The most popular varieties are undoubtedly French and English thyme. Cooks love thyme for its distinctive earthy flavor, which works fabulously with a variety of meats and vegetables. Thyme also works wonders when added to salad dressing. Healthwise, it's also a winner. In fact, its leaves are among the richest sources of potassium, iron, calcium, manganese, magnesium, and selenium.

How to Keep Herbs

To keep herbs fresher longer, wrap them loosely in a damp paper towel and put them in a plastic bag. Blow air into the bag and close it with a rubber band or a tie. You can also make an air balloon with a ziplock bag. Store them in the refrigerator for about five days.

Another option is to trim the stems and stand the herbs in water in a glass or jar. Cover them with an air-filled plastic bag and seal it with a rubber band. If you change the water daily, your herb bouquet should keep for a week in the refrigerator.

Spices

Spices can be just the thing to add pow to many dishes! Think, for example, of steak with peppercorn sauce, or curried chicken. Whether it's pepper, curry powder, hot sauce, cinnamon, nutmeg, vanilla, onion powder, paprika, or turmeric—to name but a few—spices are great go-to ingredients. Be adventurous and experiment. The idea is to keep your food interesting, and spices will do that for you! Here are just a few of my favorites.

Allspice: Native to Central and South America and used mainly in rubs for meat and poultry as well as in pickling mixtures, allspice is well named as it has a flavor similar to several spices—cinnamon, cloves, nutmeg, and black pepper—all in one. Allspice has been used as a digestive aid in traditional folk medicine for hundreds of years.

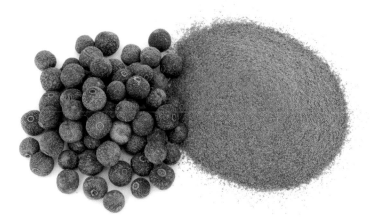

Cinnamon: You may have used it ground in baked goods, sprinkled some on your latte, or put a stick in a glass of hot apple cider. However, recent studies have shown that cinnamon may also have anti-inflammatory and antimicrobial properties and may help to normalize blood sugar levels in people with Type 2 diabetes.

Cloves give flavor to all kinds of foods, from gingerbread to bean soup, and they are traditionally used to stud baked hams. Aside from their culinary uses, however, they contain significant amounts of a compound called eugenol, which has been shown to act as an anti-inflammatory and to prevent toxicity from environmental pollutants.

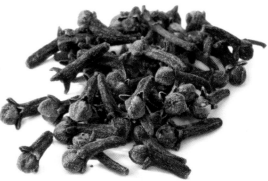

Coriander is what we call cilantro in its dried form. In studies with rats it has been shown to lower LDL (bad) cholesterol levels, and in studies of diabetic mice it has been shown to increase insulin secretion.

Cumin: In addition to being one of the spices in curry, cumin is used in many Mexican and Tex-Mex dishes, particularly to spice up a good chili. It is an excellent source of iron, and cumin seeds have traditionally been used as a digestive aid.

Curry: Although we in the West are used to buying curry in a jar or in powder form, or to ordering curry in a restaurant, in the East the term is used to designate many different kinds of spice mixtures that are individualized to the particular dish in which they are being used. For simplicity's sake, let's talk about curry powder, which generally contains, among other ingredients, turmeric, coriander, and fenugreek. Curcumin, one of the main substances in turmeric, is what gives curry its yellow color and has been shown to contain powerful antioxidant properties. (See Turmeric, below.)

Paprika can be hot or sweet, and it does a lot more than add color to your food. Traditionally known for its use in Hungarian cooking (think chicken paprikash and goulash), it contains more vitamin C than a tomato and large amounts of carotenoid antioxidants.

Pepper: There are so many different kinds, from fiery cayenne and the red pepper flakes found on the table at every pizzeria in America to the wide variety of peppercorns available in almost every supermarket. Ordinary black pepper stimulates the secretion of hydrochloric acid in the stomach, which aids digestion and is also a powerful antioxidant. Just grind your own rather than using the preground stuff on supermarket shelves. Whole peppercorns sometimes come packed in their own grinder, so you don't have any excuse!

Sea salt: As long as you're not on a sodium-restricted diet for medical reasons, sea salt is the way to go. Gram for gram it contains as much sodium as regular table salt, but because the crystals are much larger and it comes in so many varieties with such unique flavor, you may well find that you use less of it. Instead of cooking with salt, sprinkle some coarse sea salt on the finished dish to get the most flavor for the least amount of sodium.

Turmeric: Sometimes called Indian saffron, turmeric is an essential ingredient in most curries and well as chutneys—and it's what gives the mustard you get in ballparks its distinctive yellow color. The curcumin that gives turmeric its color is a powerful anti-inflammatory that studies have shown to be effective in treating arthritis.

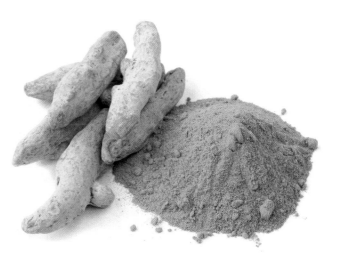

Condiments and Flavor Enhancers

All-fruit, no-sugar-added jams: My only exception to the no-jams-or-jellies rule.

Balsamic vinegar: This reduction made from grapes is not considered a wine vinegar because the grape juice, which comes from white, sweet Trebbiano grapes, is unfermented. Like wine, balsamic vinegar is aged, some for no more than 3 years, some for as long as 150 years. The older it is, the more it's going to cost. It has a sweet, smoky, slightly tart taste that is great with meats and fish as well as with fruit and cheese. And of course, use it to make your salad dressing. When buying balsamic vinegar, read the label to make sure it doesn't contain any added sugar. No need to buy the expensive stuff; it's fancier but doesn't necessarily taste better.

Bragg's Liquid Aminos: I love this stuff! It's a liquid protein concentrate, derived from soybeans, that contains many naturally occurring essential and non-essential amino acids. It tastes just like soy sauce but is gluten-free and contains no added salt. It's great in salad dressings, soups, sauces, and stir-fries, or with veggies, tofu, poultry, and fish.

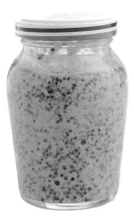

Dijon mustard: Named for its city of origin—Dijon, France—Dijon mustard is a fresh and spicy way to enhance many dishes. Made from mustard seeds, white wine, grape must (the juice pressed from grapes before fermentation), and seasonings, it's low in calories and a great emulsifier for thickening up sauces and salad dressings. Make it a staple in your Quick & Clean kitchen and brush it over chicken or fish before grilling or roasting.

Fresh salsa: Another go-to flavor booster, salsa is made from vegetables and fruits. Tomatoes, onions, green peppers, garlic, and lime juice are standard ingredients. I love it that way, but I also love mango salsa! Have fun and be creative, because this is another way to spice up your food while watching your weight. Use it as a dip for crudités, to garnish poultry, or with egg dishes. See the recipe in chapter 14.

Low-sodium soy sauce: Personally, I can't taste the difference between this and regular soy sauce. It's so flavorful that a little goes a long way. You'll find it in several of my recipes.

Nut butters: All natural, no-sugar-added nut butters make great snacks. I particularly love a sliced apple with cashew butter. Try different kinds to find the ones you like best.

Olives: Yes, I know—they're little balls of fat. But they're the same good fat you get in olive oil. Don't go overboard, but use them in moderation for their great flavor.

Must-Have Cooking Staples

These are just a few of the must-have-on-hand staples I reach for almost every day.

Low-sodium, low-fat vegetable and chicken stock or broth: Stocks and broths are flavor builders. I use them instead of water to cook grains and as a base for soups and sauces. I even use stock to sauté instead of oil. Just make sure that what you're buying is low sodium, because stocks and broths can be loaded with salt.

Cooking spray: These sprays come in many flavors. I particularly love the canola and olive oil varieties. Just be sure that what you're getting is a natural spray; some can be loaded with chemicals. You can save hundreds of calories by using them in place of butter or oil for grilling or pan-frying.

Whole wheat panko bread crumbs: When you're craving a little breaded food, panko is a good option. It's made entirely of unbleached whole wheat flour, malt extract, and a bit of salt. Use with chicken, pork, or fish to get some crunch back in your life.

Now it's time to face reality: There are some foods and drinks that are just no good for you and promise to pack on the pounds. Before we even start the Q & C fourteen-day eating plan, you *need* to know what these are.

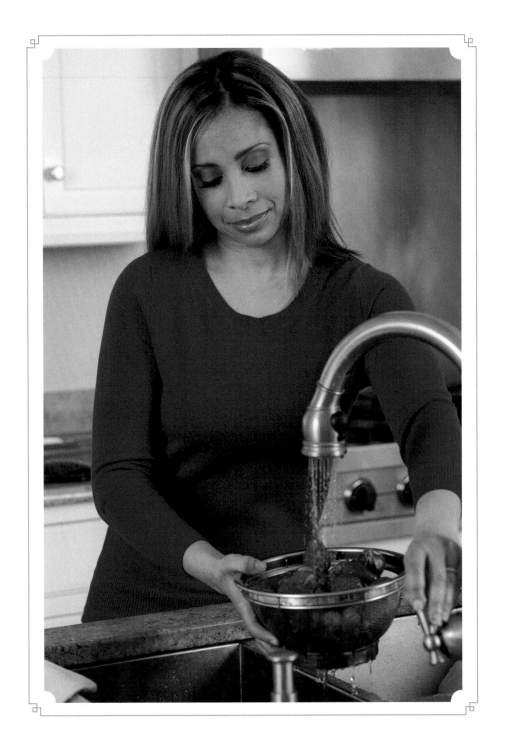

Six

Foods (and Beverages) That Can Make You Fat

Now that you know how many fabulous foods you can and should be eating on the Quick & Clean Diet, we need to talk a bit more about foods to avoid. We've talked in general about why you need to stay away from refined sugar, processed foods, and bad fat, but we haven't really discussed which foods specifically you need to avoid or cut back on eating. So that's what we're going to do now—just so there isn't any doubt.

Dry Goods

Cakes, cookies, and pies: I'm not going to tell you that you can never have another cookie or a slice of cake or pie for the rest of your life, but I also shouldn't have to remind you that these are treats to be consumed sparingly and saved for special occasions.

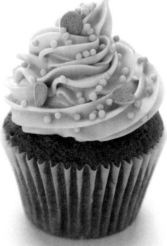

Granola: Delicious! But also high in calories and sugar. So it's not necessarily as healthy as it sounds, and is definitely not a "diet" food.

White flour (bread and pasta): When wheat is refined to make it white, the bulk of the nutrients are lost along with the bran and the germ. That's why white flour is often "enriched" in an effort to put back some of the good stuff that's been removed. But enriched or not, it turns to glucose in your body much faster than whole wheat flour, which means that it causes your blood sugar to rise—and then fall just as quickly.

White rice: Like white flour, white rice has been stripped of its nutrients, leaving only the starch, which quickly turns to sugar in your bloodstream.

Fruits

Canned fruit: Loaded with sugar and packed with preservatives, canned fruit is more like candy than fruit. Stay away from it and enjoy fresh fruits in season.

Fruit juice: Even pure juice is naturally high on the glycemic index, meaning that it raises blood sugar quickly, because it lacks the fiber in whole fruit. Eat fruit instead; if you must have juice, dilute it with water or seltzer.

Jams and jellies (except all-natural, no-sugar-added): Most commercial jams and jellies are loaded with added sugar or sugar substitutes that are just as bad for you. These are candy in a jar.

Vegetables

Canned: Aside from the fact that they're mushy and don't taste very good, most canned vegetables are loaded with salt and preservatives. Stay away from them, and if you can't buy fresh, go for frozen, with no additives. Read the label!

Meat

Canned: Hash, Spam, whatever—forget it. Too much fat and too much sodium.

Cured (bacon, ham, and hot dogs): What these meats are "cured" with is sodium nitrite. Although it was once thought to be carcinogenic, the National Academy of Sciences, the American Cancer Society, and the National Research Council all agree that there is no cancer risk from consuming sodium nitrite. That said, however, there is certainly a health risk from consuming all the sodium in these meats. So stay away from them, or at least save your hot dogs for the Fourth of July.

Luncheon meats (cold cuts): Like cured meats, these are high in sodium and also in fat. Stick with fresh white-meat turkey or chicken for your lunch.

Sausage: The problem is that you usually don't know what's in a sausage. But even if you do, it usually has more fat and salt than you should be consuming. I say stay away.

Sauces, Fats, and Oils

BBQ sauce: Forget it! This stuff is full of sugar!

Bottled salad dressings contain additives that preserve their shelf life but do nothing to preserve your health. Make your own with extra-virgin olive oil.

Ketchup: No, it's not a vegetable, no matter what the government says. And, yes, it has heart-healthy tomatoes, but also way too much sugar.

Convenience Foods

Energy bars: Have you ever really looked at the ingredients lists? They can be as long as your arm, with too many things I can't pronounce. Definitely not clean eating.

Frozen dinners are really not a good option. Even those that are labeled healthy or low cal have too many preservatives and too much sodium. Cook in batches and make your own frozen dinners at home.

Pizza: Heavy on the starchy carbs and fatty cheese, pizza is a no-no at least until you reach the Stability Stage of Quick & Clean. And then, when you do indulge, eat it sparingly, go for a thin whole wheat crust, and stay away from the meaty add-ons—oh, and no extra cheese!

Sweets

Brown sugar is a bit better than white sugar because it is less processed, but it still turns to glucose and raises blood sugar rapidly. In this case, sugar is sugar.

Candy and ice cream: Can you say empty calories? Stay away until you reach Stability, and then save these sweets for special treats.

Chocolate: Studies have shown that dark chocolate (but not milk chocolate or white chocolate) has antioxidant properties and can help to lower blood pressure. But it should still be consumed in moderation—no more than one ounce a few times a week. I'd recommend avoiding it entirely while you're trying to lose weight. You can get the same benefits from other, healthier sources.

High-fructose corn syrup (HFCS): Garbage. Fake. Corn syrup that has been processed to make it even sweeter. Research done at Princeton University has found that when rats were fed either table sugar or HFCS, those that ate the HFCS gained significantly more weight even when their total caloric intake was equal. In addition, long-term intake of HFCS caused abnormal increases in body fat, particularly in the abdominal region, and elevated triglyceride levels.

Honey (except raw): Honey has health benefits but can also raise blood sugar.

Refined sugar: What more do I need to say?

Sugar substitutes: Except for stevia and Truvia, which are all-natural herbal sweeteners, all sugar substitutes are—as their name implies—artificial. And should be avoided.

Artificial sweeteners are in just about everything—diet drinks, yogurt, pudding, ice cream, protein powders, even protein bars—so read labels carefully. Saccharin (Sweet'N Low), aspartame (Equal, NutraSweet, SugarTwin), and sucralose (Splenda) are the best-known artificial sweeteners on the market. While they might make you feel that you are making a less fattening choice, you're actually not. A study published in the *Yale Journal of Biology and Medicine* found that aspartame, acesulfame potassium, and saccharin all heightened the motivation to eat more—just like regular sugar.

Beyond weight loss, however, these sweeteners have also been linked to potential cancer risks as well as negative effects on the liver, kidneys, and other organs. They can cause headaches, gastrointestinal problems, and developmental problems in children and fetuses. Have you heard enough? I hope so.

Whipped cream: Also in the special occasion department for Stability only.

Beverages

Alcohol: Try to avoid it completely during the High Motivation Stage. Because virtually all alcohol is a carbohydrate, it turns to sugar in your body, and it also limits your body's ability to burn fat. Drinking interferes with your normal digestion because your body is trying so hard to process the alcohol that it can't properly metabolize the foods you are eating.

And of course, alcohol is nothing but liquid calories. Virtually all hard liquor has about 100 calories an ounce (that's a jigger, if you're measuring), and wine has about 100 calories in five ounces (about one glass). Twelve ounces of beer (one bottle) has around 150 calories. And then of course there are the mixers, which make it even worse.

Finally, drinking alcohol interferes with your thought process, so that the more you drink, the more you think it's okay to continue drinking—not a good idea for many reasons, among which weight loss is only one. And it also seems like a good idea to have just one more handful of peanuts or whatever other munchies are right there on the bar.

One last word about wine: You've probably heard by now that a moderate intake of red wine has a cardioprotective effect. You can thank the flavonoids in the skin and seeds of red grapes for that. Flavonoids are antioxidants that have been shown to reduce the risk of heart disease in three ways:

1. By reducing production of low-density lipoprotein (LDL)—the bad stuff.

2. By boosting high-density lipoprotein (HDL)—the good stuff—and lowering triglycerides in the blood.

3. By reducing the risk of clotting that can lead to heart attack or stroke.

So does this mean you should open the floodgates and let the red wine flow? No way! These protective properties are based on the consumption of a single five-ounce glass of wine a day for women and two for men, not a half a bottle. In fact, the very same studies show that drinking too much can negate the health benefits we just talked about and actually be harmful.

By the way, if you like red wine (and I love it!), consider this: Researchers at the University of California–Davis found that the following varieties of red wine, in the order they are listed, have the highest concentrations of flavonoids:

1. Cabernet Sauvignon

2. Petite Sirah

3. Pinot Noir

At the end of the day, it's important to use good judgment when choosing to drink at all. It is undoubtedly very much a part of our culture, and I'm certainly not condemning social drinking, but if you have a goal that you truly want to accomplish, you must change your habits. And we know that too many cocktails will sabotage all your hard work. So why would you want to do that? Just something to consider. If you do enjoy a cocktail, take a look at the Quick & Clean recipes in chapter 14.

Coffee: This is another issue on which the research findings differ. And as with alcohol, I'm discussing coffee drinking only in terms of its effect on losing weight and maintaining a healthy lifestyle. If you have any medical or other concerns, you should certainly consult a health care professional.

From all that I have read and the many doctors I have talked with, including Dr. Mehmet Oz, there is nothing wrong with that. So I'm going to say that if you want to have coffee as part of your Quick & Clean Diet plan, go ahead and have it, although I'd recommend refraining during the High Motivation Stage in order to detox your body. If I can do it, so can you. In fact, you might even get used to it and then ask yourself why you've been drinking so much coffee all these years.

Too much coffee (and how much is too much seems to vary widely from one person to another) can stimulate your nervous system, causing your adrenal gland to produce cortisol, a hormone your body releases in response to stress. That's great when you're actually in danger, because cortisol gives you the quick burst of energy you need to get out of the situation. But when the danger has passed, cortisol should dissipate and your nervous system function should return to normal. The problem with drinking coffee all day is that your cortisol levels are constantly elevated, and that's bad for your health. Chronically elevated cortisol has been shown to impair cognitive function, elevate your blood pressure, increase levels of blood sugar, and increase fat storage, particularly in the abdomen.

But here's what's tricky: A little bit of caffeine—let's say one cup of coffee, without all the added stuff (I'll get to that in a minute)—has been associated with weight loss. At least one study done by researchers in London found that subjects who consumed one hundred milligrams of caffeine (a cup has about one to two hundred milligrams) experienced a 3 to 4 percent increase in their resting metabolic rate and an 8 to 11 percent increase in energy expenditure. What that means is that, at least in the short term, you'll be burning calories faster after drinking a cup of

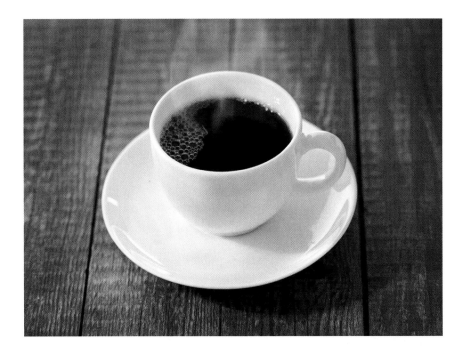

coffee. Some diet pills actually include caffeine as one of their ingredients.

Coffee is also a known diuretic, meaning that it will help flush excess water out of your body. Sounds great, but keep in mind when you get on the scale what you're losing is water, not fat, and the water loss is only temporary. In fact, it's not much different from what you'd experience if you sat in a sauna for a bit sweating and then hopped on a scale right after. The scale may indicate weight loss, but honestly, the minute you have something—anything—to drink, the fluids will be right back in your body and the number on the scale will rise again.

In addition, coffee has thermogenic properties, meaning that it produces heat and thereby takes on a fat-burning characteristic. But this isn't unique to coffee; there are plenty of other foods that have these qualities as well—for example, cayenne or chile peppers, mustard seeds, green tea, or even curry.

The problem is that the same properties of caffeine that may help you to lose some weight can cause you to become jittery and overstimulated, which is why people say they can't drink it at night, or even in the afternoon because it prevents them from getting to sleep. And several studies have shown that people who don't get enough sleep also tend to eat more and weigh more than people who do—for a variety of biochemical reasons including the fact that lack of sleep leads to increased cortisol levels, and we've already discussed the problems that can cause. In the end you need to know your own body's reaction to caffeine and let that be your guide.

Finally, let's talk about all the stuff people love to put in coffee—the cream, the sugar, the vanilla shot, the hazelnut shot, the extra milk, whatever. Those add-ons are guaranteed to make you fat. You have no chance when you start putting all those extras in your coffee. In fact, you're no longer having a morning beverage to get you going; you're actually having dessert for breakfast. And if you think you can still pull it off by using fat-free half-and-half, Splenda, and sugar-free vanilla or hazelnut flavoring, forget it. Those are nothing but unhealthy chemicals. If you can drink your coffee black, do it. If not, cut down on the bad stuff. Use less milk, used skim or low-fat milk, use light soy milk, and use stevia (see chapter 4) as your sweetener.

On a personal note . . .

I love coffee. Sometimes I crave a cup in the morning. If I do, I have it! But most of the time, I drink green tea.

Soft drinks: Nothing but chemicals. Stay away from them.

Okay, you've got the background. You've read about the various health concerns related to being overweight, and you've seen the foods you can embrace and those I want you to stay away from. Now it's time to prepare for the challenge. Ahead you will find all the guidelines you need to start the Quick & Clean Diet High Motivation Stage.

PART TWO

The Quick
& Clean Diet

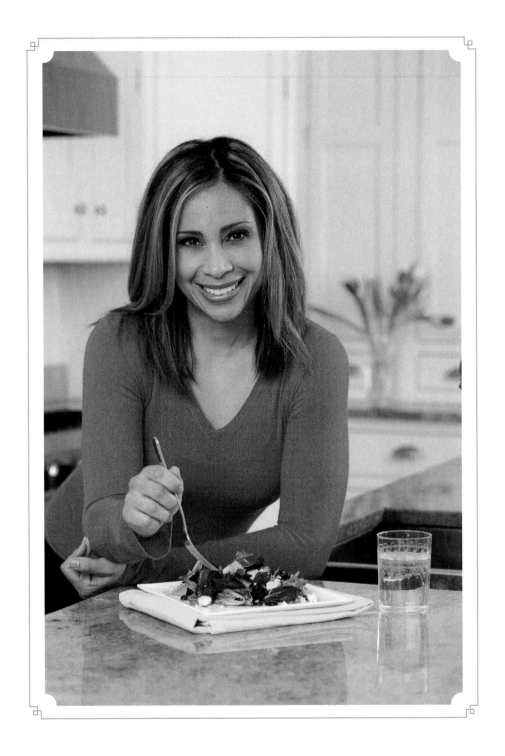

Seven

High Motivation—The Quick & Clean Fourteen-Day Challenge

The High Motivation stage is, as I've said, the most restrictive phase of the Quick & Clean Diet—but with good reason. First of all, it's when you'll get all the toxic stuff you may have been consuming for years out of your system—that's another way to look at how this can be a cleansing experience. And second, you'll see results almost right away, which is bound to keep you motivated to continue—that's the "quick" part.

By getting rid of the junk and starting to introduce good, clean food, you'll be resetting the way your body responds to what you eat. When I started my Quick & Clean adventure, I had become totally accustomed to eating foods that produced different chemical effects. Sugar would give me fast energy and a happy feeling. Caffeine gave me a buzz. Starchy carbs gave me comfort. And before I knew it, I was bouncing from sensation to sensation, and then crashing before the day was over. That is the pattern you have to break in order to lose weight. And you will!

In a few days you'll find, as I did, that you stop craving the sugar, salt, caffeine, and starch and will actually *want* to eat cleaner and lighter. I used to wake up needing coffee to get going. Not anymore. I like it, but I don't *need* coffee to get me going. I used to want something sweet or starchy in the morning. Not anymore. The High Motivation Stage helped me to change my body chemistry in order to get rid of those needs. And it happened very quickly.

Because we live in a world of instant gratification, it's tough to commit to something long-term without being able to see some sort of quick result. At least for me it is. When I don't see the result as quickly as I'd hoped, I can easily become frustrated. And that's as true for weight loss as it is for anything else. I need to know that whatever I'm doing, it's working.

I must be honest: I've always disliked the thought of having to take something away in order to gain something else, but sometimes it's necessary. To make a big change in your life, you sometimes need to focus on the greater good—and in this case that greater good is having a fit body you love (and one that loves you back) and being healthier.

So let me ask you to create this mental image: Envision two groups, those who get what they want and those who don't. In one corner you have the people who wish for it, really want to do it, dream of what it would be like, but aren't willing to do what it takes. In the other corner you have those who want it, can see it, and are willing to work hard for it. The second group gets what they want. They cross the finish line.

Part of it is determination, but the other part is structure. You must set yourself up to succeed by having a plan and sticking with it. Too many of us say we are going to do something but aren't sure exactly how we are going to achieve it. I know you know what I'm talking about. Being excited and determined to change is not enough; you must have a plan of action. Without that you just have a whole lot of intent, but no map to chart your course.

Here's the map that will get you to the end of the Quick & Clean challenge and the beginning of a whole new way of life.

The Basics

- Eat three meals a day.

- Eat lean protein, good carbs, and healthy fat at every meal.

- Have a morning and an afternoon snack every day.

- Drink water all day long.

{ *On a personal note . . .*
I never let myself get overly hungry, and you shouldn't either. It will lead to disaster! }

What's Allowed and What's Not

- Eat any vegetable *except* corn and potatoes. If you want to add additional steamed or grilled vegetables to any meal, do so.

- *Limit* legumes to ¼ cup in a salad once a week.

- Eat any fruit *except* bananas, cherries, mangoes, and pineapples.

- Eat any of the dairy products listed in chapter 4.

- Eat any of the proteins.

- Eat any of the fats.

- Use any of the herbs, spices, and condiments in the Quick & Clean pantry (chapter 5).

{ *On a personal note . . .*
I've seen diets that don't allow you to eat any fruit. For me, that's just ridiculous. I love fruit, and I need it. I don't believe there is any reason to cut it out of your life completely. On this diet you will always be able to eat fruit. The ones to avoid during the High Motivation Stage are those that are highest in sugar. But don't worry: You'll be welcoming them back into your life very soon! }

- Have no more than 2 teaspoons of agave syrup a day. Have as much stevia or Truvia as you like.

- Have a cup of coffee in the morning if you wish, but have it with skim or low-fat milk.

- Do *not* eat any grains.

- Do *not* drink any alcoholic beverages

Before You Begin

Go through your pantry, fridge, and freezer and get rid of all the food you have on hand that will make you fat. You may think this is an extravagant thing to do but, believe me, it's worth it. If it isn't there, you won't be tempted by it, and in the end isn't the point to make this process as easy as possible?

It's worth looking through the meal plan that follows and stocking up on staples before you start the program. Also, make as many dishes as possible in advance. That way you'll know you have them on hand when you get hungry and won't have any excuse to "cheat."

You can use the menus on the meal plan exactly as they're written or substitute your own favorite clean dishes. You can switch days, switch combinations, or repeat a favorite dish as often as you like. Just be sure that you use only the ingredients allowed on this stage of the diet. Please remember that I have included nutritional information merely as a reference for anybody who needs to know; this should not be your focus. If you do find yourself very hungry—or you feel like you are not getting enough

On a personal note . . .

Some nutritionists say that lunch should be your biggest meal of the day, because it's eaten during the time when you're most active. If that works for you, great, but I think it really depends on your lifestyle. I've worked nights for many years, so the evenings are my most active time. And for many of us, "dinner" is also a time for socializing. So I say it's up to you. If you want to switch the lunch and dinner meals during any stage of Quick & Clean, please feel free to do so. The goal is to make you comfortable and, therefore, successful.

calories—apples, peanut butter, almond butter, and almonds are always healthy options for adding sustenance. If these don't appeal to you, choose another healthy option that's Q & C approved. Just remember, this is not an excuse to eat a big fat cheesy pizza!

Also, look through chapter 14 to find additional High Motivation recipes that are not included in the meal plan, and feel free to use those too.

Make a pitcher or two of flavored waters and keep them in the fridge. You can also decant them into bottles to carry with you throughout the day. To make flavored waters, place the fruits of your choice in a mesh tea ball steeper and immerse it in a pitcher of water. Let it steep for several hours; when it's as "fruity" as you desire, remove the tea ball. Or just put the cut-up fruit in the pitcher and strain it out when the water is flavored to your taste. Feel free to mix and match different fruits—I like strawberry-raspberry and strawberry-kiwi water, for example.

Water with Fruit

Remember, you can drink unlimited amounts of water and green tea. If you are sensitive to caffeine, buy caffeine-free green tea. I drink it in the afternoon. Or you can drink herbal tea if you hate the taste of green tea. Rooibos tea is another good option that's very good for you and has no caffeine. Dr. Oz loves it! It will help you feel full. Vegetable portions are also unlimited. They will also help make you feel satisfied.

Day One

Breakfast
Q & C Super Protein Smoothie (p. 140)
Hot green tea

Snack
20 raw almonds
½ pink grapefruit sprinkled with Truvia
Glass of strawberry water

Lunch
Tarragon Chicken Salad (p. 166)
Glass of water with orange slice

Snack
Strawberry Greek Yogurt Parfait (p. 202)
Glass of raspberry water

Dinner
Shrimp Taco Lettuce Wraps (p. 177)
Glass of orange water

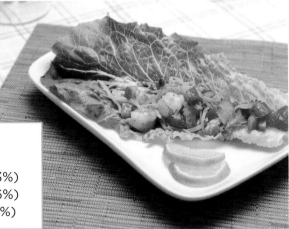

Analysis for Day 1:	
Calories	1060
Total Fat	38 g (43%)
Carbohydrates	70 g (26%)
Protein	118 g (31%)

Day Two

Breakfast
Turkey and Tomato Omelet (p. 149)
Green tea

Snack
14 raw almonds
6 ounces whole vanilla yogurt
    sprinkled with cinnamon
Glass of lemon water

Lunch
Chopped Greek Chicken Salad (p. 175)
Glass of orange water

Snack
20 fresh or frozen grapes
Glass of strawberry water

Dinner
Rosemary Dijon Chicken Breast
    over Steamed Spinach (p. 181)
Glass of lime water

Analysis for Day 2:	
Calories	1204
Total Fat	59 g (30%)
Carbohydrates	84 g (27%)
Protein	92 g (43%)

On a personal note . . .

I suggest having green tea every morning because it is loaded with antioxidants that have been linked to everything from fighting cancer to preventing heart disease. In addition, one study reported in *The American Journal of Clinical Nutrition* found that people who consumed green tea extract experienced a significant increase in their energy expenditure (that is, the rate at which they burned calories) as well as their rate of fat oxidation (the process by which fat is converted into usable energy). At least one other study conducted on obese people in Thailand also supported these conclusions.

Day Three

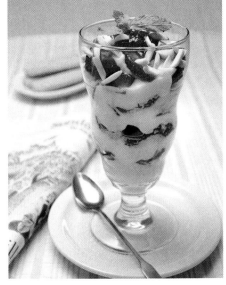

Breakfast
Crustless Spinach Quiche (p. 146)
Green tea

Snack
Strawberry Greek Yogurt Parfait (p. 202)
Glass of lemon water

Lunch
Q & C Grilled Scallop Salad
   with Basil Vinaigrette (p. 169)
Glass of lime water

Snack
2 tablespoons almond butter
   with 5 baby carrots
Glass of lemon water

Dinner
Olive Oil Herb-Roasted Flank Steak (p. 183)
Steamed Spinach with Lemon (p. 198)
Glass of raspberry water

Analysis for Day 3:	
Calories	1087
Total fat	60 g (47%)
Carbohydrates	64 g (23%)
Protein	87 g (30%)

Day Four

Breakfast
Santorini Omelet (p. 157)
Green tea

Snack
½ cup mixed berries
6 ounces whole vanilla yogurt sprinkled with cinnamon
Glass of lemon water

Lunch
Grilled Shrimp and Cannellini Bean Salad (p. 170)
Glass of lime water

Snack
20 fresh or frozen grapes
15 raw almonds

Dinner
Garlic Lime Chicken on a Bed of Steamed Spinach (p. 192)
Glass of lemon water

Analysis for Day 4:
Calories	1120
Total Fat	50 g (26%)
Carbohydrates	101 g (35%)
Protein	75 g (39%)

Day Five

Breakfast
Peaches and Cinnamon Cream Smoothie (p. 141)
Green tea

Snack
20 fresh or frozen grapes

Lunch
Tarragon Chicken Salad (p. 166)
Glass of lime water

Snack
10 raw almonds

Dinner
Salmon with Snow Peas
    and Fresh Dill (p. 190)
Glass of strawberry water

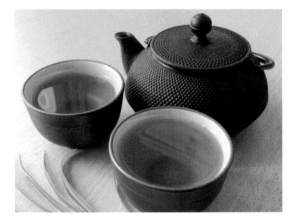

Analysis for Day 5:	
Calories	1325
Total Fat	45 g (33%)
Carbohydrates	132 g (38%)
Protein	114 g (29%)

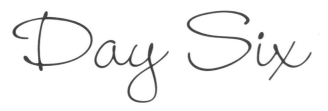

Day Six

Breakfast
Strawberry Greek Yogurt Parfait (p. 202)
Green tea

Snack
1 small pear with 2 small pieces of farmer's cheese
Glass of raspberry water

Lunch
Creamy Chicken Salad (p. 174)
Glass of lime water

Snack
15 baby carrots with 2 teaspoons cashew butter
20 raw almonds
Glass of lemon water

Dinner
Grilled Pork Chops with Red Onion Apple Relish (p. 195)
Steamed Spinach with Lemon (p. 198)
Glass of strawberry water

Analysis for Day 6:	
Calories	1004
Total fat	40 g (35%)
Carbohydrates	78 g (30%)
Protein	91 g (35%)

Day Seven

Breakfast
Scrambled Eggs with Pico de Gallo (p. 153)
Green tea

Snack
$1/2$ cup mixed berries
6 ounces whole vanilla yogurt
   sprinkled with cinnamon
Glass of lemon water

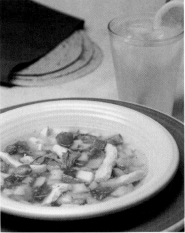

Lunch
Mexican Soup (p. 176)
2 wedges Laughing Cow Light
   Creamy Swiss Cheese
Glass of orange water

Snack
15 baby carrots with 1 tablespoon
   cashew butter and Ranch Dip (p. 204)
Glass of strawberry water

Dinner
Chicken Marsala (p. 182)
Steamed Broccoli Rabe with Lemon (p. 198)
Glass of lime water

Analysis for Day 7:	
Calories	1074
Total fat	45 g (30%)
Carbohydrates	97 g (34%)
Protein	84 g (36%)

Day Eight

Breakfast
Q & C Super Protein Smoothie (p. 140)
Green tea

Snack
10 raw almonds

Lunch
Chopped Greek
    Chicken Salad (p. 175)
Glass of lemon water

Snack
6 frozen grapes

Dinner
Sautéed Shrimp with Arugula and Tomatoes (p. 196)
Steamed Spinach with Lemon (p. 198)
Glass of lemon water

Analysis for Day 8:	
Calories	1039
Total fat	39 g (34%)
Carbohydrates	50 g (19%)
Protein	121 g (47%)

Day Nine

Breakfast
Old-Fashioned Eggs and Bacon (p. 161)
Green tea

Snack
½ cup mixed berries
Glass of lemon water

Lunch
Creamy Chicken Salad (p. 174)
Glass of lime water

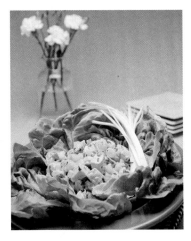

Snack
15 raw almonds

Dinner
Q & C Grilled Chicken Kebabs (p. 185)
Steamed Broccoli Rabe with Lemon (p. 198)
Glass of raspberry water

Analysis for Day 9:	
Calories	1031
Total fat	40 g (43%)
Carbohydrates	64 g (24%)
Protein	114 g (33%)

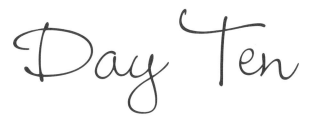

Day Ten

Breakfast
Strawberry Greek Yogurt Parfait (p. 202)
Green tea

Snack
10 raw almonds
Glass of strawberry water

Lunch
Tarragon Chicken Salad (p. 166)
Glass of lime water

Snack
½ cup 2 percent cottage cheese
    with 1 teaspoon agave syrup
Glass of orange water

Dinner
Salmon with Snow Peas
    and Fresh Dill (p. 190)
Glass of lemon water

Analysis for Day 10:	
Calories	1017
Total Fat	41 g (35%)
Carbohydrates	69 g (26%)
Protein	102 g (39%)

Day Eleven

Breakfast
Santorini Omelet (p. 157)
Green tea

Snack
Creamy Strawberry Cottage Cheese with Almonds (p. 205)
Glass of lemon water

Lunch
Grilled Chicken, Tomato,
  and Arugula Salad (p. 168)
Glass of lime water

Snack
Red pepper slices with
  Ranch Dip (p. 204)

Dinner
Super-Clean Shrimp and
  Broccoli (p. 178)
Glass of raspberry water

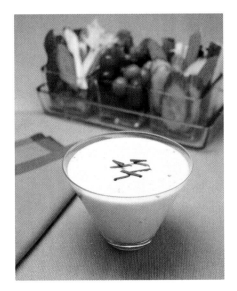

Analysis for Day 11:
Calories   1068
Total fat   42 g (35%)
Carbohydrates   38 g (14%)
Protein   138 g (51%)

Day Twelve

Breakfast
Q & C Super Protein Smoothie (p. 140)
Green tea

Snack
10 raw almonds

Lunch
Shrimp Taco Lettuce Wraps (p. 177)
Glass of lime water

Snack
Small pear with 2 slices of farmer's cheese

Dinner
Rosemary Dijon Chicken Breast
  over Steamed Spinach (p. 181)
Glass of orange water

Analysis for Day 12:
Calories   1043
Total Fat   40 g (34.5%)
Carbohydrates   64 g (24.5%)
Protein   107 g (41%)

Day Thirteen

Breakfast
Strawberry Kefir Smoothie (p. 143)
Green tea

Snack
15 raw almonds
Glass of lemon water

Lunch
Q & C Grilled Scallop Salad
   with Basil Vinaigrette (p. 169)
Glass of orange water

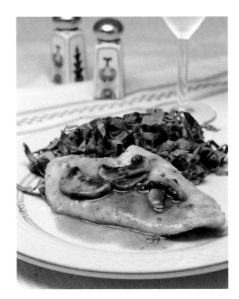

Snack
2 tablespoons cashew butter
   with 15 baby carrots
Glass of lime water

Dinner
Chicken Marsala (p. 182)
Steamed Spinach with
   Lemon (p. 198)
Glass of lemon water

Analysis for Day 13:	
Calories	1001
Total fat	43 g (36%)
Carbohydrates	94 g (35%)
Protein	75 g (28%)

Day Fourteen

Breakfast
Q & C Super Protein Smoothie (p. 140)
Green tea

Snack
½ cup 2 percent cottage cheese with 1 teaspoon
   agave syrup
Glass of orange water

Lunch
Creamy Chicken Salad (p. 174)
Glass of lemon water

Snack
1 small pear with 2 teaspoons
   cashew butter
Glass of strawberry water

Dinner
Olive Oil Herb-Roasted
   Flank Steak (p. 183)
Steamed Broccoli Rabe
   with Lemon (p. 198)
Glass of lime water

Analysis for Day 14:	
Calories	1116
Total fat	34 g (28%)
Carbohydrates	64 g (23%)
Protein	137 g (49%)

You got through it! Now breathe a sigh of relief! That's why it's called a challenge—but now you're in a better place for it. Now you move on to the next stages: Grounding, where you will continue to lose weight, and then Stability, the place you want to be. Take a look at the guidelines in the next chapter, and remember to enjoy the process.

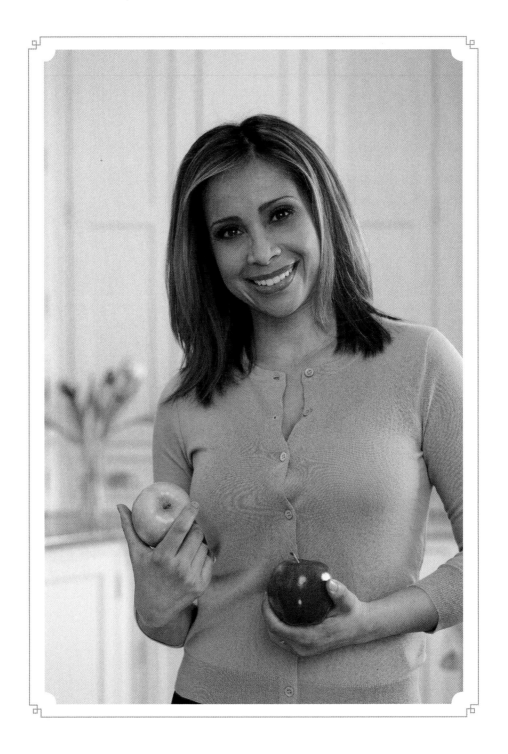

Eight

Stages Two and Three— Grounding and Stability

In this book I have included recipes you can use in the Grounding and Stability Stages of the Quick & Clean Diet—a time when of course you can continue to use any recipes from the High Motivation Stage— but there are no specific meal plans for these stages. The reason is that both stages are open-ended. You'll be staying on the Grounding plan until you reach your goal weight, and how long that takes will depend on how much you have or want to lose. Next comes the Stability Stage, when you should no longer be thinking of this as a "diet." Once you reach your weight loss goal, you'll have made the Quick & Clean way of eating your lifestyle for the rest of your life! You'll know what you can and can't eat to maintain your weight; you will have found which foods you like and don't like; and, hopefully, you'll have developed a repertoire of Quick & Clean dishes of your own. In other words, you won't need me to tell you what you should or shouldn't be eating anymore.

Grounding

Notice anything? Do your clothes fit better? Do you feel hopeful about getting into your favorite old jeans very soon? Or maybe you already can! At this point you should be feeling better overall. You've just spent two weeks correcting your eating habits and clearing your body of toxins. Your cravings should be gone, and you're *wanting* to eat healthy foods. I know that at the end of the first fourteen days, I was feeling pretty good. I was more in control of my eating habits. I didn't crave all the salty or sugary foods I had in the past. I was sleeping better and had more energy.

I still wanted and needed to lose more weight, but there were a few foods I was missing. That's how the Grounding Stage of the diet evolved. At this point you can reintroduce a small quantity of good grains into your life.

If you want a piece of whole grain toast with breakfast, fine. A whole wheat wrap for lunch? Great. Just stay away from the refined, processed white stuff—no going back to Wonder Bread, if that's what you were eating before. For me, my new toast was a slice of Food for Life Ezekiel Bread with cashew butter.

What about some brown rice with dinner? Why not? You can even have pancakes if you want.

But your metamorphosis is hardly over. In this Grounding Stage you will continue to lose weight, but most likely at a more gradual pace. There's nothing wrong with that. In fact, having a wider range of healthy foods in your diet will help you stick with the plan. Being too restrictive for too long is simply too difficult for most people. Stay with this stage until you reach your goal weight. Then move on to Stability.

DURING THE GROUNDING STAGE YOU WILL:

- Continue to eat all the foods you did during the fourteen-day challenge.

- Continue to avoid corn and potatoes.

- Continue to limit legumes.

- Continue to avoid bananas, mangoes, cherries, and pineapple.

- Continue to avoid all alcohol.

- Add back ½ cup of any grain on the Foods to Love list (chapter 4) or 1 slice of whole grain bread per day.

- Have 1 or 2 alcoholic drinks or glasses of wine a week, if you like (and by that I do mean no more than 2!).

Stability

You're there! You've reached your goal weight. Congrats! Now you can focus on maintaining what you've achieved for the rest of your life. I hope you feel good, because you've worked hard and that little bit of sacrifice was worth it. Those dream jeans fit. Go out and get that slinky strapless dress you've been wanting, because it will look great on you, and you deserve a reward for giving yourself the greatest gift there is: a dynamite body and much better health.

Your body should respond to foods differently. Like me, you may taste certain things you used to love and think they are much too sweet or much too salty. And you probably like the way your butt looks a lot more than you like the doughnuts at the coffee shop down the street. Now, when you think of a snack, think of one that's Quick & Clean—maybe a few frozen grapes or an apple with cashew butter.

At this point you can eat any of the Foods to Love (chapter 4), including all the grains. Just remember that portion size still counts. No matter how healthy a food is, when you overeat you're going to become overweight.

Drink wine or alcohol in moderation, but remember, it's still empty calories!

Don't see this stage as an invitation to throw everything you've just worked for out the window. It's important to reflect on how hard it was to get here and how important it is to stay here—not just because you love the way you look, but because you care about your health. Don't throw it all away by returning to those bad habits.

See this segment as an opportunity to really experiment with healthy foods. Keep broadening your food base so you never get bored.

PART THREE

Quick & Clean Strategies to Ensure Your Success

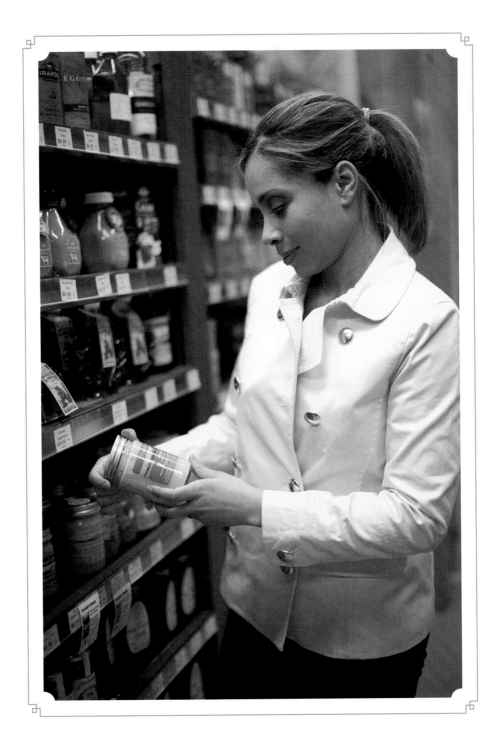

Nine

Quick & Clean Food Shopping Strategies

Michael Pollan said it best in his book *In Defense of Food: An Eater's Manifesto:* "Today there are thousands of other edible food-like substances in the supermarket." Foods manufactured in factories make all sorts of alluring claims about how they've been "enhanced" to improve your health. Really? Think about that. Why would a manufactured food product be more beneficial than a natural, unadulterated whole food filled with vitamins, minerals, and other nutrients—not to mention flavor?

But all those "enhanced" and tempting foods can make a trip to the grocery store overwhelming and potentially dangerous to your health and your waistline. I've fallen for their allure and into the trap of shopping by those glossy circulars more than once, so here are a few tips based on my own hard-won experience to help you navigate the aisles.

Never go food shopping when you're hungry: If you're like me, going to the grocery store hungry is like committing diet suicide. Forget it! If you're famished, it's too hard to resist those things you would normally be able to talk yourself out of buying.

Never go without a list: You have to be ready to nip temptation in the bud, and to do that you need a plan. Without that list, the deli counter, the bakery, the prepared foods section, the snack center, and everything on sale will be sucking you in. But if you can walk into that store knowing exactly what you need to buy, you won't start wandering aimlessly. Check out the store's circular online so you know what's on special before you get there. I do it all the time.

Avoid the interior aisles as much as possible: I know I've talked about this before, but it's worth repeating. Sure, there are things you'll need to buy in those aisles—just be wary. Stick with exactly what's on your list.

Beware of the serving size: When you do buy something packaged, such as whole wheat pasta, brown rice, or sugar-free jam, make sure you read the label—especially the part at the top that says "serving size" and "servings per container." A food can look relatively low in calories until you realize that the "calories per serving" are only for a quarter or less of the entire package.

Think about Going Organic

There are numerous arguments for going organic: It is better for the environment, produces safer and often tastier food, and is kinder to animals, to name just a few. But for now, let's just focus on what it does for you.

Organic foods are grown (and in the case of animals, fed) without the pesticides used in conventional farming. Those pesticides have been shown to be toxic to humans, and the fewer of them you have in your system, the better off you will be, especially if you have any concerns about having children. Some pesticides found in conventionally grown foods have been shown to reduce fertility rates in women. Many of them have also been shown to be carcinogenic in large quantities. The problem is that we are exposed to so many chemicals—in the water, in the soil, and in the air—that we don't really know how many are in our bodies. I think it's best to avoid consuming them whenever possible.

That said, organic foods are generally more expensive (although you can now find them at many of the price clubs and big-box stores), so you may want to determine which foods to buy organic when you can. Personally, I start with milk and eggs. Most conventional milk is filled with antibiotics, artificial hormones, and pesticides, so if you or your children drink milk regularly, going organic would be a great place to begin. The same is true of eggs, because of the antibiotics fed to conventionally raised chickens.

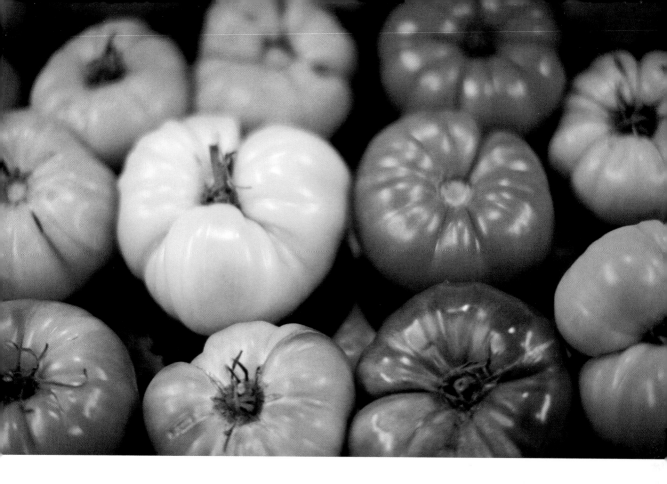

As for the chickens themselves, if you can't go organic, try for free-range. At least free-range chickens spend some of their time grazing and eating worms (what they're supposed to eat). A study done by researchers at Pennsylvania State University found that eggs from grazing chickens have twice as much vitamin E, 40 percent more vitamin A, and three times as many omega-3s as conventionally grown eggs.

And of course, the same would hold true for organic, grass-fed cattle. When I eat beef, that's what I buy.

When it comes to fruits and vegetables, the Environmental Working Group provides yearly lists of what they call the Dirty Dozen and the Clean Fifteen. The Dirty Dozen are those that are most likely to contain the most pesticides. They are (in order, starting with the worst):

THE DIRTY DOZEN

Peaches	Cherries
Apples	Kale
Sweet bell peppers	Lettuce
Celery	Imported grapes
Nectarines	Carrots
Strawberries	Pears

The Clean Fifteen are either those that have thicker skins (and are, therefore, less likely to absorb pesticides) or those we peel before eating. They are (starting with the best):

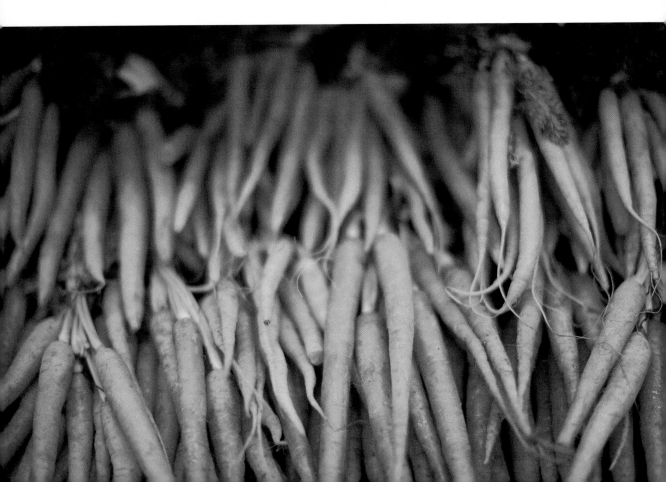

Onions	Asparagus	Papaya
Avocados	Sweet peas	Watermelon
Sweet corn	Kiwis	Broccoli
Pineapples	Cabbage	Sweet potatoes
Mangoes	Eggplant	Tomatoes

If you're deciding which produce to buy organic, start with the Dirty Dozen!

Go Local

Another way to eat well is to buy foods grown in your area. Why should you buy strawberries from California if you live in Michigan and there is a grower in your state? The strawberries closest to you will undoubtedly be fresher than those that have to travel hundreds of miles to your grocery store, and you will also be supporting your local farmers.

Buy Seasonal

If you buy foods when they are in season, you will find that they are generally more flavorful. And as they will be plentiful, they will also be less expensive. Historically, before refrigerated trucks and foods shipped by air, our ancestors ate both locally and seasonally. It's fun and exciting to see fresh asparagus arrive in season, or to get really sweet corn and wonderful tomatoes at your local produce market or farm stand.

So far we've talked about a lot of different foods, some more expensive than others. But your new eating plan should never challenge your budget. There are many ways to eat well while also minding your money . . .

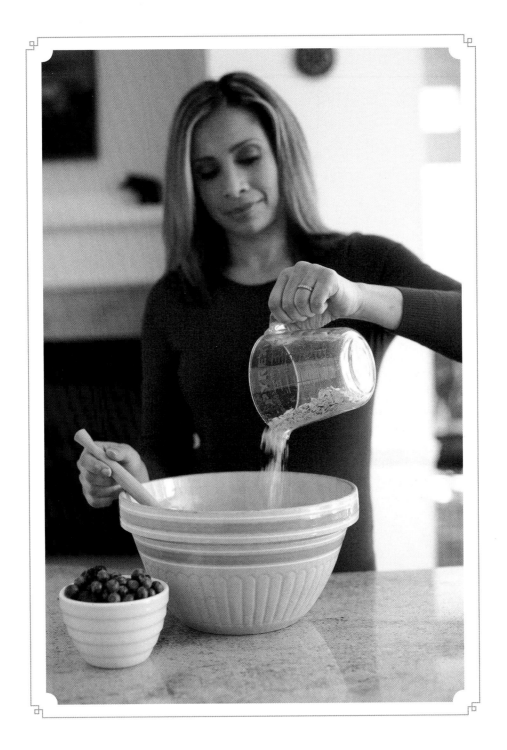

Ten

Cheap Eats

There is no reason why you should have to break the bank in order make better food choices. It is true that food is far more expensive than it was ten years ago, and healthy foods can be more expensive than some junk foods, but if you stop buying the junk you didn't need in the first place, you'll have more food dollars to spend on the good stuff.

And there is good news on the food horizon. In the past several years, price clubs and big-box stores have been carrying more and more good fresh foods. These days Costco, Sam's Club, BJ's, Walmart, and Target are about much more than just stocking up on canned goods and cleaning supplies. You can go there to buy fresh foods affordably. And you can even stock up on all-natural frozen meats and vegetables. If you haven't got a lot of storage space, try going with a friend and sharing.

Farmers' markets are another great option. Take a walk around and see all the variety there is on offer: not just fresh fruits and vegetables but also eggs, meat, poultry, and fish. Not to mention the jars of fresh honey, all-fruit jams, nut butters, pickles, oils, and 100 percent whole-grain pasta and bread along with artisanal cheeses!

Also, if you possibly can, I urge you to grow your own vegetables and herbs—even plant a fruit-bearing tree (if you have the space) or plant strawberries in a pot. Use a part of your yard, or plant on a terrace, a porch, or a deck. If nothing else, grow some herbs on your windowsill. When you grow your own, there is no question about whether or not the food has been treated with pesticides, whether it has been previously frozen, or when it was picked. You alone can be the master of what you put in your mouth. Besides, it is really gratifying to watch your food grow and then pick your own string beans, broccoli, lettuce, tomatoes, zucchini, strawberries, or even apples from your own backyard. And if you have children, it's a great way to teach them about nutrition and how foods grow. I'm lucky enough to have an apartment with a terrace, and that's where I plant. I admit that planting, growing, and harvesting take work, but in the end (and if the weather cooperates) you will have some of the best produce you can eat. You'll be able to prepare it simply too, because the better the quality of the food, the less you need to do to it. You may find yourself eating as you pick—especially vegetables like string beans or tomatoes. Talk about gratifying; there's no better way to eat!

So, when you're trying to save, remember:

Shop the price clubs and big-box stores: You can find good-quality foods, even organic, in these stores because they buy in bulk and can extend the value to you.

Buy frozen: Yes, your first choice should be fresh, but if you can't find fresh, buy frozen. It's cheaper, and it allows you to stock up.

Get an extra freezer: If you can afford it and have the space, an extra freezer in your basement or garage will allow you to grab all the best stuff when it's on sale. You can also freeze your own produce at the end of the growing season.

Shop circulars: It's a great idea to stock up when things are on sale. Just beware of buying what you don't need, even though it's tempting. I know; I've done it myself.

Leave your credit cards at home: If all you have to spend is the cash in your pocket, you won't be able to spend more.

Don't throw it out: When you're done with a meal, don't you dare throw anything out. If it can be a leftover, have it tomorrow. If you can turn it into soup, sauce, or dog food, wrap it up. There is no time or money to waste. So if you can have a meal for tomorrow on hand, for yourself of someone else in your family, do it. And don't forget about people who are in need. You can drop extra food off at pantries or even a park bench. I never leave a restaurant without a doggie bag, because I know that, even if I'm not going to eat it myself, I can give it to someone in need.

Eat eggs: They're cheap and nutritious. You've heard the saying, "Eggs are the perfect food." They're packed with protein, and if you're concerned about cholesterol, you can use just the whites. Add peppers, onions, or any vegetable and you have a nutritious meal. Who doesn't love breakfast for dinner?

Frozen fish right out of the freezer case at the grocery store is perfectly fine and inexpensive. Just choose fillets that are plain (no sauce added), and prepare them however you like. It's a great way to eat lean and cheap.

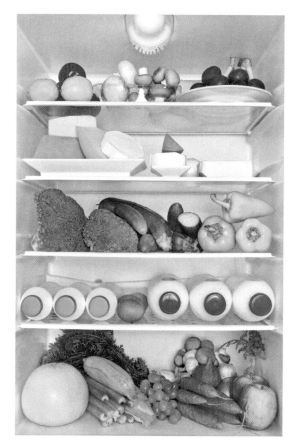

Ground turkey meat: These days you can find ground turkey that is over 90 percent fat-free, and it's very inexpensive. If you add some vegetables, sauté everything in a bit of olive oil, and stuff it in a whole wheat wrap, you can feed the whole family a healthy meal quickly and without breaking the bank.

Cook seven on Sunday: Cook once a week and have meals on hand. I do it on Sunday afternoons while the kids are out playing. I've found that by having precooked meals in the refrigerator or freezer, I'm less likely to make unscheduled trips to the market or be tempted to order something in at the last minute. In the end, it saves me both time and money.

So you've got the food; now let's take a look at ways to prepare it. You'll be surprised by how various cooking techniques allow you to keep the calories low and the taste great. Let's explore them!

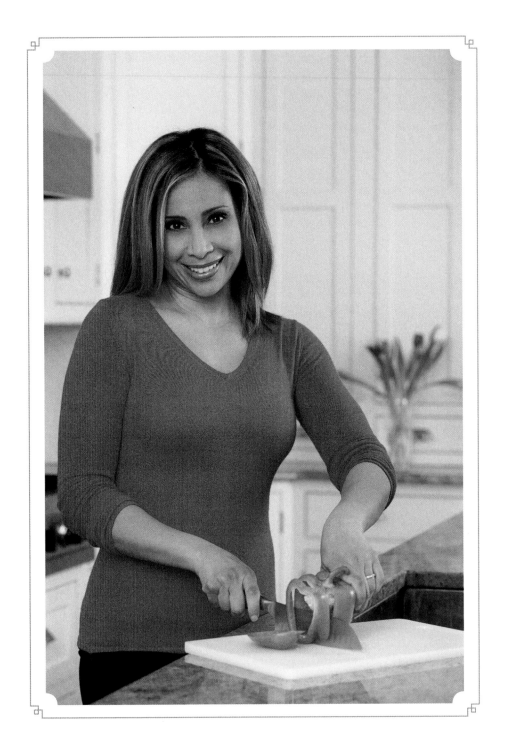

Eleven

Quick & Clean Cooking Techniques and Restaurant Rules

Assuming that you won't be hiring a personal chef anytime soon, the best way to take control of your eating is to cook for yourself. I'm not suggesting that you take a course at the Cordon Bleu or become a contestant on the next season of *Top Chef,* but if—like many Americans—you've been eating most of your meals out, you'll need to master a few of the techniques used in the recipes I provide. I'm not suggesting that you never go to a restaurant again—in fact, we'll be talking about that in this chapter as well. The recipes aren't difficult, and once you've mastered them, you'll be able to make any number of quick, healthy meals for yourself and your family.

When you're using good, fresh ingredients, simplest is often the best. Quick & Clean cooking works because it doesn't require a lot of preparation or a long list of fancy ingredients. The idea is never to be hungry, so I don't want you to be bogged down slaving in the kitchen.

Lean Cooking Techniques

One of the simplest ways to make your food leaner is to prepare it in a healthy manner. That's why I'd like to walk you through some of the most slimming cooking methods. You can refer to these techniques when preparing the recipes in this book or invent new ones of your own.

Steaming is a form of "wet cooking" used primarily for vegetables, fish, and chicken, and is about as clean as it gets. Steaming helps retain most of the vitamins and minerals that are often lost when proteins or vegetables are cooked directly at high temperatures.

You will notice that steamed foods also retain their gorgeous, natural bright color and crisp texture.

To steam food you will need a metal steam basket, a pot with steam holes, or an inexpensive bamboo basket. Fill a saucepan with about an inch and a half of water. Place the steam basket in the saucepan (making sure that it doesn't become submerged in the water)

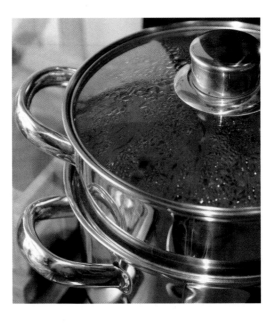

and bring the water to a boil. When the water is boiling, place food in the steam basket and cover the pot with a tight-fitting lid. Depending upon the food, steaming should take only a few minutes, because the steam is so hot. When food is bright in color and tender, it is done. If you are cooking vegetables, be sure they are still somewhat crisp; you don't want mushy vegetables.

Poaching: This very delicate way to prepare foods keeps the flavors and aromas from breaking down during the cooking process. There are so many great things about poaching: It's very quick, it requires no added fat, you can add herbs and/or broth or stock to the poaching water for extra flavor, and you don't need any special equipment. All you need is a basic saucepan and you're ready to go. Poaching is great for delicate proteins like fish, but it also works well with chicken. You will notice that poaching leaves foods with a kind of silky finish.

To poach, place your ingredients in a saucepan and add water. Bring the liquid to a boil and reduce the heat to a simmer. Food is done when it is firm and opaque.

Grilling: Simple and so tasty! Grilling is an American pastime, but it also can be a low-fat, flavorful way to cook. Dry heat from the grill smokes and sears the food. Don't you love those grill lines? And here's what's so great: The fat actually melts off the meat and drops to the bottom of the grill; whatever is left can be easily trimmed. Marinades, rubs, and brines are all great ways to kick up the flavor of grilled food. Don't forget that grilling is not just for meat and poultry: Fish, vegetables, tofu, even fruit all work great on the grill.

Stir-frying is a tasty way to prepare foods quickly. A key cooking method in Asian countries, it has become an American favorite as well. Unlike deep-fat frying, or breading and frying, stir-frying uses very little fat, and the food is constantly moving in the pan so it doesn't sit in fat while it's cooking. One thing to remember is that the foods that take longest to cook should be added to the pan first, followed by those that cook more quickly. Stir-frying is a great option for vegetarian meals, and you shouldn't feel that you need to go out and buy a wok in order to try it. Any skillet set over high heat will work just as well. The trick is to keep stirring!

Roasting takes longer than the cooking methods above; still, after you put the food in the oven it doesn't need much tending, so you can just go about your other business while it cooks. Roasting is the process of dry-heat cooking that basically uses hot air to dry your food. It's delicious because this method of cooking allows the natural juices and added spices to concentrate,

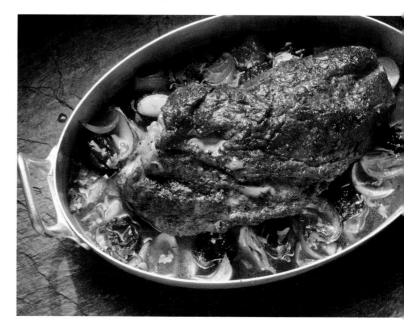

which brings out the full flavor in meat, poultry, fish, and vegetables. It leaves food tender on the inside and crisp or caramelized on the outside. Temperatures depend on the density of the food that you are cooking, and recipes will indicate set temperature, but it's usually at least 300 degrees or hotter.

Restaurant Rules—How to Survive Eating Out

It would be unrealistic to think that you can always eat at home or bring prepared food with you wherever you go—besides, sometimes it's fun to eat out. But you need to be armed with some guidelines so you don't sabotage everything you've worked for. And I don't know about you, but when I'm trying to lose a few pounds, eating in restaurants makes me nervous.

I have a hard time passing up all those tasty-sounding foods on the menu, especially when whomever I'm with seems to be ordering with abandon and eating everything in sight. Well, now neither one of us has to think that way anymore, nor do we have to feel anxious about going out to eat. I have thought this through for both of us, and I believe my suggestions will work for you as they have for me. The next time you go to a restaurant, consider these strategies:

Don't go famished: That's simply setting yourself up to fail. Foods that normally wouldn't tempt you will now taunt you because you're ravenous! Don't put yourself in that position. Instead of "saving up" your calories by skipping your afternoon snack, eat the snack. The whole point of having snacks on the meal plan is to keep you from becoming too hungry—ever. That's the point. Then go to the restaurant as a rational human being, not a crazed diet fiend.

Read the menu in advance: Almost every restaurant has a website, and almost every website includes menus, so check it out. If you know what you're going to eat before you get there, you'll be much less likely to succumb to temptation.

Nix the bread: Even if you're at a stage when you can have a slice or two of whole wheat bread, confronting that bread basket is just too tempting. If your dinner companion agrees, just ask the waitperson not to leave it on the table. Or, if the person you're eating with does want some bread, ask him or her to put a slice or two on a bread plate and then ask the waiter to remove the basket.

Ask to have it your way: You can always ask to have something steamed or broiled without butter or oil instead of sautéed or fried. You can ask to have extra vegetables instead of potatoes. You may already be asking to have your salad dressing "on the side," and this is just one more request you can make to avoid diet disaster. I've found that it's very rare for a chef or a restaurant not to accommodate any reasonable request.

Take it to go: You're not a child anymore, and you don't have to belong to the clean plate club. Most restaurant portions are much larger than those we would make for ourselves at home, which is one of the dangers of eating in restaurants. So by all means ask for a doggie bag, whether or not you have a dog. And if you think looking at all that food will be too tempting, ask your server to wrap some of it up before you even begin. Or split an entree with your dining companion. Many restaurant meals are definitely big enough for two. I want you to go home feeling satisfied, not stuffed or as if you need to be rolled out the door.

By now you've agreed to make a change in your life. While you're in this mind-set, let's talk about exercise. It should never be overwhelming, so don't overthink this. I'm just talking about movement—something, anything. Let's take a look at simple things you can do.

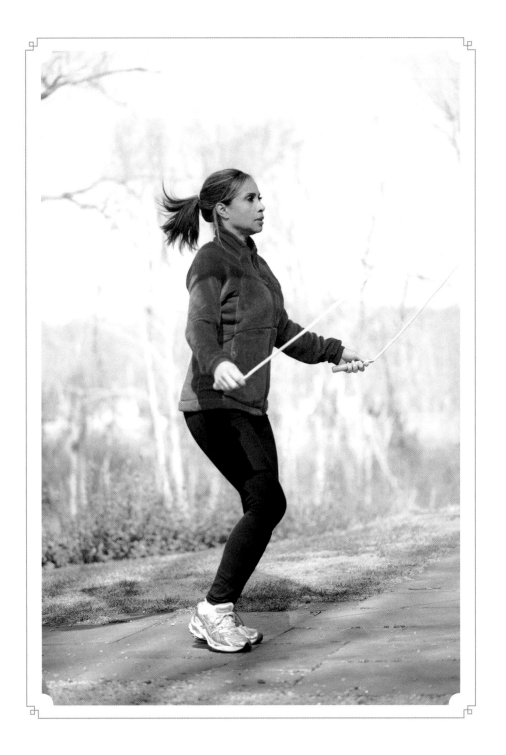

Twelve

Get a Move On

I have some friends who absolutely hate to exercise, and others who cannot go a day without hitting the gym. For most of my life, I'd say I fell somewhere in the middle. Then I had kids. Now I simply have to figure out a way to exercise every day. Of course it's important for my health and my body, but it also does wonders for my head.

I can't be your personal trainer, but you need to figure out a way to move your body—if possible every day. Most health professionals say you should exercise for at least thirty minutes seven days a week. That would certainly be great, but if you can't, do what you can. You may well find that the more you do, the more you want to do, especially when you start to see and feel the results.

What It Does

On the simplest level, the more you move, the more weight you will lose. Remember that calories are units of energy, and the more energy you expend the more calories you burn. When you burn more than you consume, you win because you lose!

In terms of health, there is absolutely no doubt anymore that exercise is good for your heart, your lungs, and your blood pressure—to name just the most obvious health benefits of working out. And once your heart and lungs are working better, you'll have more energy to do all the things you have or want to do (including sex). Exercise doesn't tire you; on the contrary, it peps you up.

Weight-bearing exercise also strengthens your bones and joints and builds lean muscle tissue—and muscle burns calories faster than fat. I'm not talking here about bench-pressing two hundred pounds. Just pick up a couple of handheld weights (at whatever weight you can manage) and lift your arms over your head. Studies have shown that weight training done on a regular basis can help prevent osteo-porosis and even help to rebuild bone already lost. In addition, building lean muscle helps to improve your balance and coordination so that you are less likely to fall and injure yourself.

In addition, many studies have shown that exercises helps to relieve stress and improve your mood by releasing chemicals in the brain called endorphins—the ones associated with what is often called the runner's high. Some research has even shown that exercise can help to treat at least some forms of clinical depression. In a randomized controlled trial by researchers at Duke University, depressed adults who participated in an aerobic exercise program did as well as those treated with the antidepressant drug Zoloft. That doesn't mean Zoloft doesn't work; it just means that getting your butt moving can be a really cheap and effective drug.

Finally, exercise has been shown to promote better sleep, particularly in sedentary adults. Makes sense. If you feel better and are less stressed, you're going to sleep better. And we've already discussed the fact that lack of sleep can lead to weight gain—not to mention irritability.

What to Do

As I said, I'm not a personal trainer—yours or anyone else's. But here are a few tips I can pass along based on my own experience and the information I've gathered. None of this is rocket science, but it makes good sense and it's worth repeating.

- If you can join a gym, do it. Not only will you have access to professional equipment and professional advice, but I've found that if you pay for something, you're that much more likely to use it. Maybe join a Spinning class. You may find that it's addictive.

- If there's a sport you enjoy, figure out how and where you can do it. Tennis? There are many indoor courts you can use in the winter, and many parks have courts where you can play in the summer. Swimming? Find a pool. Skating (ice or roller)—find a rink. Or try something new. When you enjoy doing something, it's no longer a chore; it's fun. And if you can find a friend to do it with, so much the better.

- Find an exercise buddy. Many studies have shown that people who exercise with another person are much more likely to keep it up—due to mutual encouragement or the competitive spirit, or just because they know someone else is counting on them to show up.

- If you do nothing else, get out and walk. I live in the city, so I tend to walk a lot. In fact, research has shown that city dwellers on the whole tend to walk much more than those who live in the suburbs or the country, where the farthest walking distance is often from the door to the car. In good weather, look for a park. When it's nasty (or very hot), try an indoor mall—just leave your cash and credit cards at home. Years ago, when I was living in Davenport, Iowa, I used to see people walking the mall in the middle of winter when it was around zero degrees outside. At first I had no idea what they were doing; I learned they were "mall walkers"—people who got their daily exercise by indoor walking, particularly in extreme temperatures. I thought it was brilliant! Safe, climate-controlled, and stimulating.

- I'm sure you've all heard about parking farther from your destination or taking the stairs instead of the elevator, so do it.

- Be realistic. If you make a plan that's too ambitious or that doesn't fit your lifestyle, you're not going to keep it up. If you've never walked farther than the corner, don't plan on starting with five miles. If you hate to get up, don't plan on setting the alarm an hour earlier—do your exercise at lunchtime or after work.

- Remember that any movement is exercise. That means running around with your kids, cleaning the house, planting a garden, mowing the lawn, walking the dog—anything that gets you moving.

- Finally, if you've never done any exercise before—or in the last ten years—do consult a health professional before you start any new routine.

Bottom line: Physical activity is a great way to feel better, gain health benefits, and have fun.

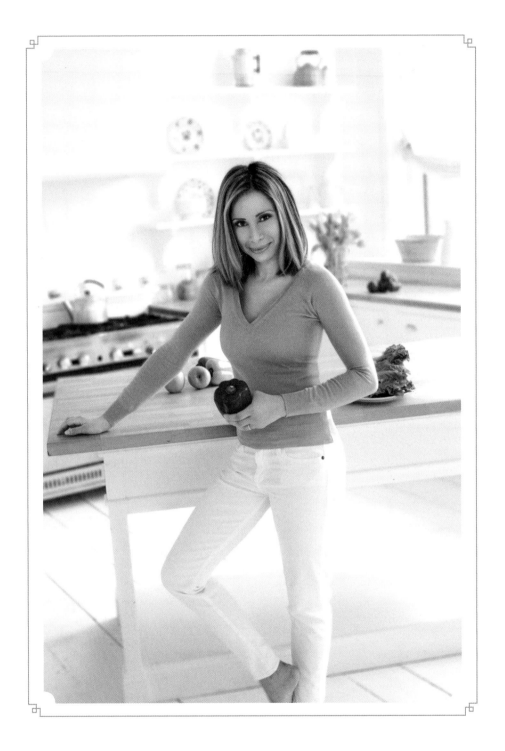

Thirteen

Last Words

Just a few last words before I send you on your way.

First of all, bravo to you for wanting to change and coming this far. For that alone you should celebrate yourself. It may not be easy, and you may not be perfect every moment of every day. I'm certainly not. But what I discovered was that every time I walked away from temptation or took on a new challenge, it got easier the next time, and it will for you too. You can do this.

One of the most important things to remember as you move forward is to be kind to yourself. If you beat yourself up before you get started, you are guaranteed to fail. It just won't work. So do me a favor: Start this with a positive attitude, and visualize what it's going to be like when you succeed—how you'll look, how you'll feel. Keep that image in the forefront of your brain every time you hit a bump or have a moment of doubt. I guarantee that the desire to succeed will outweigh your desire for a cookie. Maybe not every single time, but certainly most of the time. And don't let one cookie get you down. Eating a cookie does not mean you've failed. It just means you need to not eat the next cookie.

When you hear that inner voice saying *You can't, you've never succeeded before so why should this time be different*—and you *will* hear it from time to time; I did—just tell it to be quiet. That's trash talk; don't give it any power. It's nothing but a tape that's been playing over and over in your head, possibly for years. Break it! Burn it! Throw it away! It no longer applies! You have the power now. And I'm right there, holding your hand in spirit. So let's prove your doubting-self wrong!

Now it's time to learn how to cook for each stage of the Quick & Clean Diet. Ahead you will find recipes for all the dishes on this diet. If you don't like something, feel free to substitute a different vegetable or protein. Just make sure it's on the Foods to Love list.

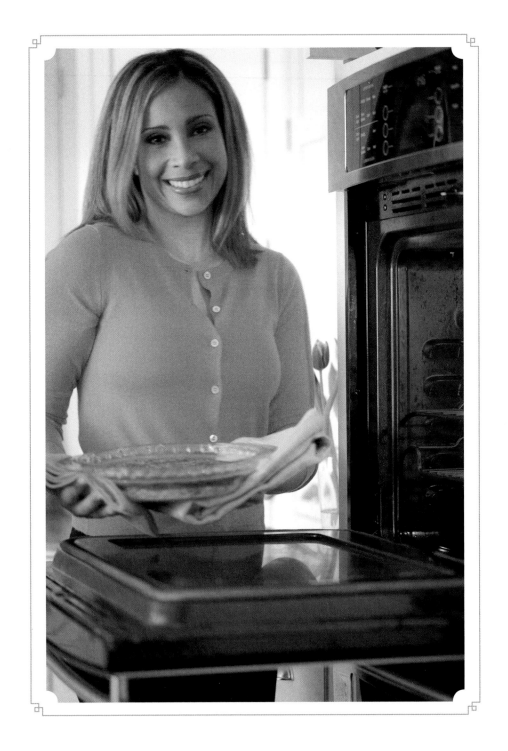

Fourteen

Recipes for Every Stage of the Quick & Clean Diet

If you like food, this is the fun part! Think about taking pleasure in preparing everything you eat. It's part of the process. While you should eat until your body is satisfied, don't set out to overeat. If a dish looks like it's for more than one meal, take your portion and save the rest for another day.

This chapter includes recipes for all stages. You will find the following icons next to the recipe title indicating the stage for which they are appropriate:

HMS—High Maintenance Stage

GS—Grounding Stage

SS—Stability Stage

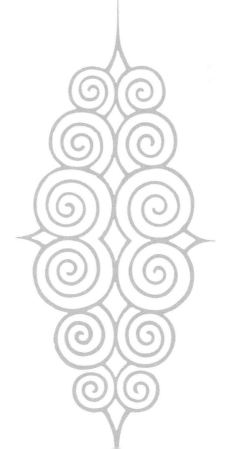

Breakfast

Q & C Super Protein Smoothie

HMS, GS, SS

Some people may be concerned about consuming uncooked egg whites, but when they are pasteurized there is no reason to worry. This is one of my favorites because it tastes great and is very filling.

MAKES 1 SERVING

6 ounces pasteurized liquid egg whites
1 scoop vanilla protein powder
½ cup fresh or frozen berries of your choice
1 packet Truvia
Handful of ice cubes

Place all the ingredients in a blender and whirl for 1 minute or until smooth.

Per serving: Calories 249; total fat 2 g; saturated fat 1 g; cholesterol 70 mg; sodium 328 mg; carbohydrates 12 g; dietary fiber 3 g; sugars 6 g; protein 42 g

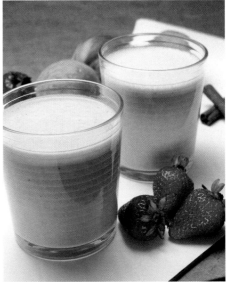

Peaches and Cinnamon Cream Smoothie

HMS, GS, SS

This may be a breakfast smoothie, but it tastes like dessert.
In the summertime I love to make it with fresh peaches. If
you don't like soy milk, feel free to use almond milk or even 2
percent fat cow's milk.

MAKES 1 SERVING

1½ cups cut-up fresh or frozen peaches

2 cups unsweetened vanilla soy milk

1 cup 2 percent fat Greek yogurt

2 teaspoons agave syrup

1 teaspoon vanilla

½ teaspoon ground cinnamon

Handful of ice cubes

Combine all the ingredients in a blender and whirl for 1 minute
or until smooth.

Per serving: Calories 445; total fat 9 g; saturated fat 3 g; cholesterol 15
mg; sodium 255.5 mg; carbohydrates 61 g; dietary fiber 6 g; sugars 38 g;
protein 34 g

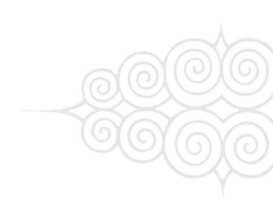

Mixed Berry Flaxseed Oil Super Smoothie

HMS, GS, SS

This is a great way to get some essential oils in your diet. Feel free to use a variety of berries.

MAKES 1 SERVING

$\frac{1}{2}$ cup blueberries

$\frac{1}{2}$ cup strawberries

2 teaspoons flaxseed oil

2 teaspoons dark agave syrup

1 cup 2 percent fat Greek yogurt

2 cups unsweetened rice milk

1 teaspoon vanilla extract

Handful of ice cubes

Combine all the ingredients in a blender and whirl for 1 minute or until smooth.

Per serving: Calories 577; total fat 19 g; saturated fat 4 g; cholesterol 15 mg; sodium 227 mg; carbohydrates 80 g; dietary fiber 3 g; sugars 47 g; protein 23 g

Strawberry Kefir Smoothie

HMS, GS, SS

MAKES 1 SERVING

4 large strawberries, fresh or frozen
6 ounces unsweetened plain kefir
1 packet Truvia
5 ice cubes

Combine all the ingredients in a blender and whirl for 1 minute or until smooth.

Per serving: Calories 86; total fat 0 g; saturated fat 0 g; cholesterol 3.5 mg; sodium 85.5 mg; carbohydrates 15 g; dietary fiber 3 g; sugars 8 g; protein 8 g

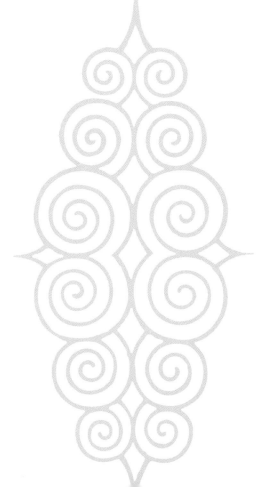

Strawberry Breakfast Parfait with Slivered Almonds

GS, SS

This recipe may have the word *breakfast* in it, but I love to eat it any time of day. In the morning it will give you great energy.

MAKES 1 SERVING

6 ounces 2 percent fat plain Greek yogurt
1 teaspoon vanilla extract
1 packet Truvia
1 cup fresh strawberries
2 tablespoons all-fruit apricot preserves (no sugar added)
1 tablespoon slivered almonds

1. Combine the yogurt, vanilla, and Truvia.

2. In a tall glass, create alternating layers of yogurt and strawberries, starting with the yogurt. Finish with a layer of strawberries, top with the apricot preserves, and sprinkle with the almonds.

Per serving: Calories 229; total fat 7 g; saturated fat 2.5 g; cholesterol 11 mg; sodium 51 mg; carbohydrates 31 g; dietary fiber 4 g; sugars 15 g; protein 17 g

Q & C Fresh Salsa

HMS

Salsa is amazingly helpful when watching your weight. It tastes great, and it's very low in calories. I put it on everything: in salads, over chicken, on vegetables and plain scrambled eggs! Be creative with salsa.

MAKES ABOUT 4 SERVINGS

> 4 medium-size ripe tomatoes
> ¼ cup minced red onion
> 1 garlic clove, chopped
> 1 teaspoon sea salt
> ¼ cup fresh cilantro leaves
> 1 teaspoon chopped jalapeño (optional)

Combine all the ingredients in a food processor and pulse until coarsely chopped. Keep leftovers refrigerated in an airtight container.

Per serving: Calories 26; total fat 0 g; saturated fat 0 g; cholesterol 0 mg; sodium 397 mg; carbohydrates 6 g; dietary fiber 2 g; sugars 4 g; protein 1 g

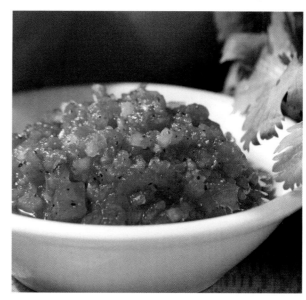

Crustless Spinach Quiche

HMS, GS, SS

This dish can be made in advance and stored in the refrigerator tightly covered for up to three days. Leftovers can also be refrigerated so that you can simply cut off a portion and have it for breakfast. It's also great as a snack, for lunch, or with a side salad for dinner. Eat it at room temperature, or reheat it for a few minutes in the oven, or quickly in the microwave.

MAKES 8 SERVINGS

1 tablespoon canola or safflower oil
½ cup minced onion
1 (16-ounce) package frozen spinach, thawed and squeezed dry
8 large eggs, preferably organic
½ cup 2 percent fat cottage cheese
½ teaspoon ground nutmeg
¼ cup grated Parmesan cheese

1. Preheat the oven to 350°F.

2. Heat the oil in a medium saucepan. Sauté the onion until soft and translucent.

3. Add the spinach and cook for three minutes. Remove from the heat. Drain excess liquid.

4. Combine the eggs, cottage cheese, and nutmeg in a small bowl, add the spinach, and mix.

5. Transfer to a 9 x 13-inch nonstick baking dish and bake in the preheated oven for 30 minutes. When done, the center will remain moist.

6. Dust with the Parmesan, cut, and serve.

Per serving: Calories 130; total fat 8 g; saturated fat 2 g; cholesterol 190 mg; sodium 211 mg; carbohydrates 5 g; dietary fiber 2 g; sugars 1.5 g; protein 11 g

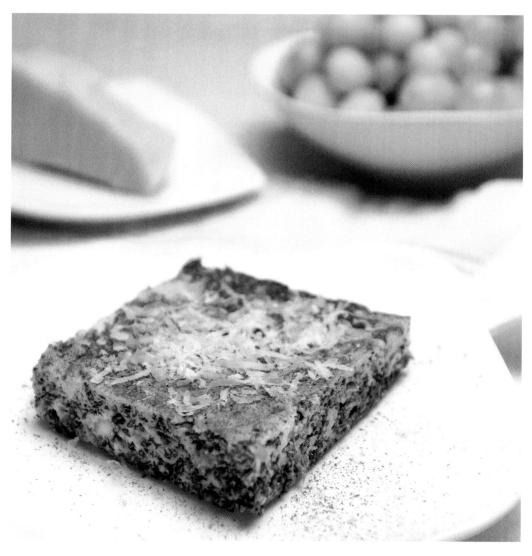

Smoked Salmon and Spinach Frittata
GS, SS

This is such a decadent breakfast that it makes me feel like I'm eating brunch. It will keep, covered, in the refrigerator for up to 3 days, or you can cut it into individual portions and freeze it.

MAKES 8 SERVINGS

1 tablespoon canola oil
½ cup finely chopped onion
1 cup baby spinach leaves or 16 ounces chopped frozen spinach, thawed
8 large eggs, preferably organic
½ cup 2 percent fat cottage cheese
¾ cup freshly grated Parmesan cheese
4 ounces smoked salmon, cut in bite-size pieces

1. Preheat the oven to 350°F.

2. Heat the oil in a medium skillet and sauté the onion and spinach until wilted. Drain well and set aside.

3. In a bowl, whisk together the eggs, cottage cheese, and Parmesan. Stir in the salmon and the spinach mixture.

4. Pour into a 9-inch pie plate sprayed with nonstick spray and bake for approximately 45 minutes, or until the quiche is set.

Per serving: Calories 150; total fat 10 g; saturated fat 3 g; cholesterol 197 mg; sodium 355 mg; carbohydrates 3 g; dietary fiber 0.5 g; sugars 1 g; protein 14 g

Turkey and Tomato Omelet

HMS, GS, SS

This one is really easy and fast to make. Feel free to add more tomatoes, scallions, or onions if you like.

MAKES 1 SERVING

2 eggs, preferably organic
1 teaspoon chopped scallion or onion
2 tablespoons chopped tomato
Pinch of sea salt
Freshly ground pepper to taste
1 slice nitrite-free turkey breast

1. In a small bowl, whisk together the eggs.

2. In a separate small bowl, combine scallion, tomato, salt, and pepper

3. Heat a skillet sprayed with nonstick cooking oil. When the skillet is hot but not smoking, add the eggs.

4. Lay the turkey on top and add tomato and scallion mixture. Fold when the eggs are cooked. Sprinkle with more pepper if you like.

Per serving: Calories 163; total fat 10 g; saturated fat 3 g; cholesterol 381 mg; sodium 408 mg; carbohydrates 2 g; dietary fiber 0 g; sugars 1 g; protein 16 g

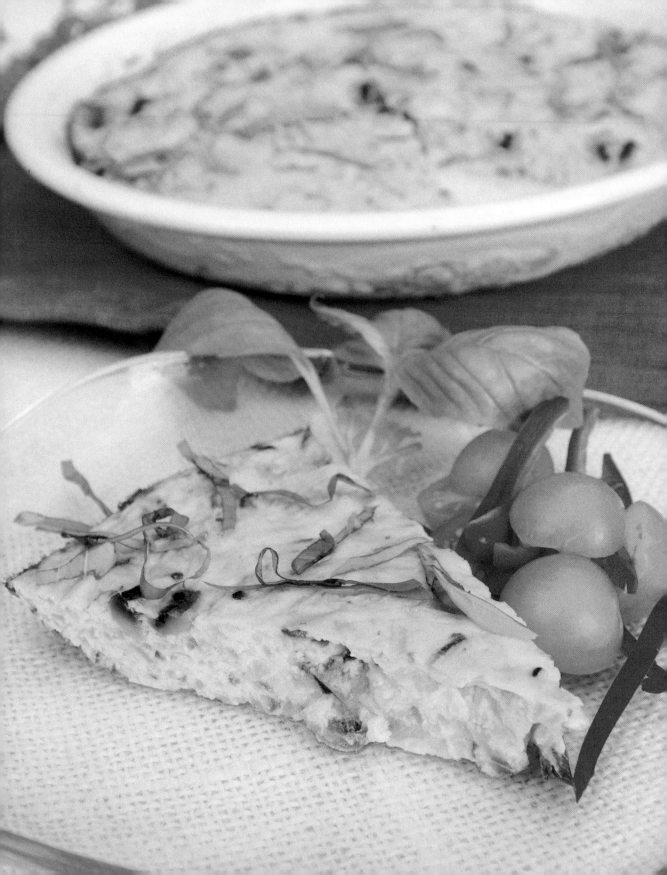

Zucchini Frittata

HMS, GS, SS

This is a nice alternative to an omelet or quiche. It's packed with vegetables and protein and will keep in the refrigerator for up to 3 days. Alternatively, you can cut it into individual portions and freeze.

MAKES 6 SERVINGS

1 tablespoon canola oil
3 cups grated zucchini
½ cup sliced mushrooms
1 cup chopped onion
3 eggs, preferably organic
½ cup skim milk
¼ cup chopped fresh basil

1. Preheat the oven to 350°F.

2. Heat the oil in a medium skillet. Add the zucchini, mushrooms, and onion and sauté, stirring, until softened.

3. Remove from the skillet, drain, pat dry, and let cool a little.

4. In a bowl whisk the eggs with the milk, and add the vegetables. Transfer to a 9 x 13 nonstick baking dish or a 9-inch pie dish. The pie dish should be sprayed with nonstick cooking spray if it's glass.

5. Cook for 40 minutes or until the center of the frittata is firm but not dry. Sprinkle with the basil, cut into slices, and serve.

Per serving: Calories 80; total fat 4 g; saturated fat 1 g; cholesterol 93 mg; sodium 50 mg; carbohydrates 6 g; dietary fiber 1 g; sugars 4 g; protein 5 g

Steel-Cut Oatmeal with Vanilla Protein and Strawberries

GS, SS

This is a creamy, comforting hot breakfast for a cold winter morning, or anytime!

MAKES 1 SERVING

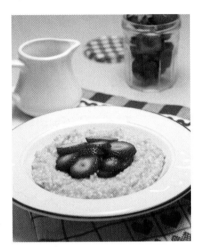

¼ cup steel-cut oatmeal*
½ scoop vanilla protein powder
¼ cup hulled and sliced strawberries

1. Cook the oatmeal according to package instructions.

2. When done, stir in the protein powder and top with the strawberries. You can also add a little skim milk to make it even creamier.

Per serving: Calories 222; total fat 4 g; saturated fat 1 g; cholesterol 35 mg; sodium 25 mg; carbohydrates 31 g; dietary fiber 5 g; sugars 3 g; protein 17 g

---

* **Note:** Steel-cut oats generally take much longer to cook than other types of oatmeal, but you can now find quick-cooking steel-cut oats in the market. If you're in a hurry, try them. They are not as nutritious as the steel-cut oats that take 30 minutes to cook, but they're better than the instant oatmeal you buy in stores.

Scrambled Eggs with Pico de Gallo

HMS, GS, SS

Quick and satisfying! Use as much of the pico de gallo as you like.

MAKES 1 SERVING

¼ cup chopped tomato
¼ cup chopped onion
1 tablespoon chopped fresh cilantro
1 tablespoon fresh lime juice
2 eggs, preferably organic

1. Combine the tomato, onion, cilantro, and lime juice. Set aside.

2. Whisk the eggs together in a small bowl.

3. Spray a nonstick skillet with cooking spray and set over medium heat. Add the eggs and scramble to your desired doneness.

4. Serve with the pico de gallo mixture sprinkled on top or on the side.

Per serving: Calories 183; total fat 10 g; saturated fat 3 g; cholesterol 372 mg; sodium 259 mg; carbohydrates 9 g; dietary fiber 1 g; sugars 3 g; protein 14 g

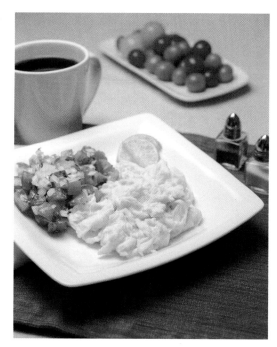

Super-Fast Breakfast Tacos

GS, SS

A taste of the Southwest. Try this when you want to spice things up.

MAKES 1 SERVING

3 eggs, preferable organic
1 (10-inch) whole wheat tortilla
Q & C Fresh Salsa (recipe on page 147)

1. Spray a medium skillet with nonstick cooking spray and heat to medium.

2. Whisk the eggs together in a small bowl and warm the tortillas. When the pan is heated, scramble the eggs to your desired doneness.

3. Fill the tortillas with the scrambled eggs and top with the salsa.

Per serving: Calories 401; total fat 19 g; saturated fat 6 g; cholesterol 558 mg; sodium 756 mg; carbohydrates 32.5 g; dietary fiber 4 g; sugars 1 g; protein 24.5 g

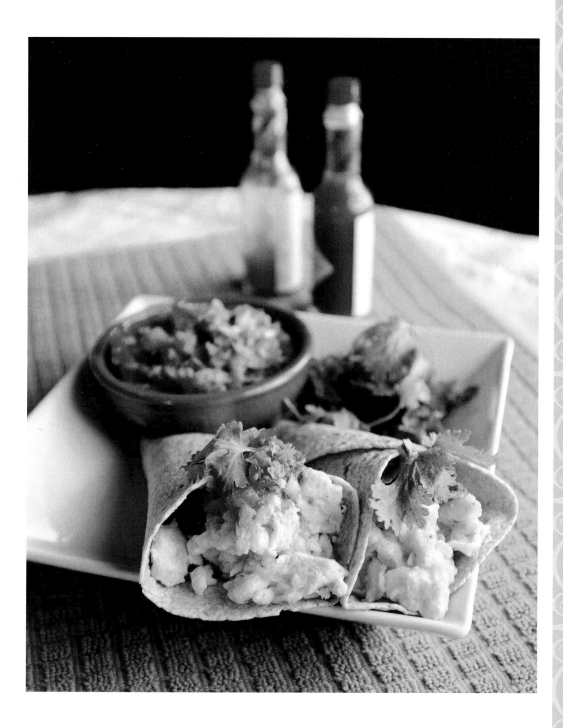

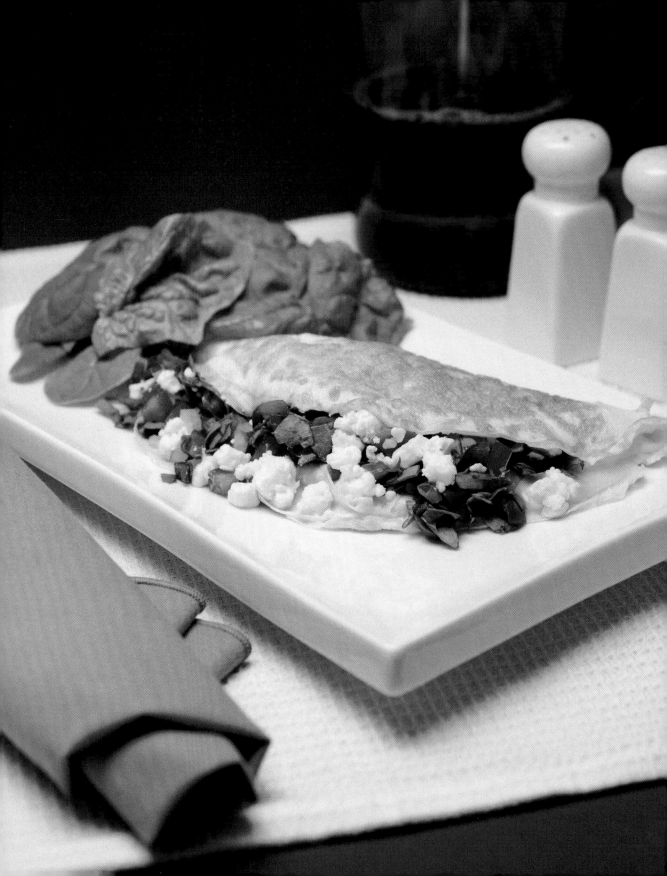

Santorini Omelet

HMS, GS, SS

This omelet has a lot of flavor and texture, which is why it's one of my favorites. Sometimes I even eat it for lunch!

MAKES 1 SERVING

> 2 tablespoons chopped red onion
> 2 tablespoons chopped tomato
> 2 tablespoons chopped black kalamata olives
> 1/4 cup chopped fresh spinach
> 2 eggs, preferably organic
> 1 tablespoon crumbled feta cheese

1. Spray a small skillet with olive oil cooking spray and set it over medium heat.

2. Add the onion, tomato, olives, and spinach. Sauté for two minutes or just until softened. Remove from the pan and set aside.

3. Remove the skillet from the heat, wipe it clean, spray again, and reheat.

4. Whisk the eggs in a small bowl and add them to the reheated pan.

5. When the eggs begin to set, spoon the reserved tomato-and-onion mixture onto one side of the omelet, and sprinkle with the cheese. Slide a spatula under the empty side of the omelet and fold it over. Let the cheese melt for a minute and serve.

Per serving: Calories 198; total fat 13 g; saturated fat 4 g; cholesterol 378 mg; sodium 375 mg; carbohydrates 5 g; dietary fiber 1.5 g; sugars 2 g; protein 15 g

Country Chicken-Apple Sausage and Egg White Scramble

HMS, GS, SS

I usually make this on weekends when I have time to really enjoy a long breakfast, but you can have it any day of the week. Look for all-natural, additive-free sausage, available at many markets.

MAKES 1 SERVING

¼ cup thinly sliced scallions
1 tomato, diced
2 chicken-apple sausages, diced in squares
1 cup baby spinach leaves
4 egg whites, whisked
Sea salt and freshly ground pepper to taste

1. Spray a medium skillet with olive oil cooking spray and set it over low heat.

2. Add the scallions and let them soften a bit, then add the tomato. Add the sausage and cook for 3 minutes. Add the spinach and let it wilt. Remove from the heat and set aside.

3. Spray a second skillet with nonstick cooking oil spray and set it over medium heat. Add the egg whites and scramble until they're cooked the way you like them.

4. Toss with the sausage mixture, sprinkle with salt and pepper, and serve.

Per serving: Calories 233; total fat 5.5 g; saturated fat 2 g; cholesterol 50 mg; sodium 789 mg; carbohydrates 18 g; dietary fiber 3.5 g; sugars 13 g; protein 29 g

Q & C Thyme-Infused Shrimp and Eggs

HMS, GS, SS

The aroma of fresh thyme is so great,
and it's such a wonderful complement
to the shrimp, that this feels like a
gourmet meal without all the fuss.

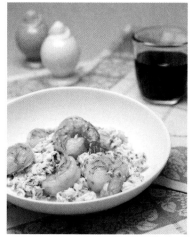

MAKES 1 SERVING

> 2 teaspoons extra-virgin olive oil, divided
> 6 uncooked medium shrimp, cleaned and
>   deveined
> 4 egg whites
> Leaves from 1 sprig fresh thyme
> 1 tablespoon chopped chives
> 2 teaspoons low-sodium soy sauce
> Sea salt and freshly ground pepper to taste

1. Spray a skillet with olive oil cooking spray and add
   1 teaspoon of the olive oil.

2. Set the pan over medium heat, add the shrimp, and sauté
   until slightly pink.

3. Whisk together the egg whites, thyme, chives, soy sauce, and
   the remaining teaspoon of olive oil in a bowl, then add to
   the shrimp in the pan.

4. Fold with a rubber spatula, breaking up and lightly fluffing
   the eggs. When the shrimp are bright pink and the eggs no
   longer runny, remove from the heat, season with salt and
   pepper, and serve.

Per serving: Calories 181; total fat 8 g; saturated fat 1 g; cholesterol 64
mg; sodium 876.5 mg; carbohydrates 3 g; dietary fiber 0 g; sugars 1 g;
protein 24 g

Cinnamon Oat Protein Pancakes with Strawberry Agave Sauce

GS, SS

This is a tasty breakfast to make on weekends or when you have extra time and need a treat.

MAKES 2 SERVINGS

For the sauce:

5 strawberries, hulled and halved

2 tablespoons water

1 tablespoon dark agave syrup

For the pancakes:

4 large egg whites

$\frac{1}{2}$ cup 2 percent cottage cheese

$\frac{1}{2}$ cup oatmeal

$\frac{1}{2}$ teaspoon baking powder

$\frac{1}{4}$ teaspoon ground cinnamon

1. To make the sauce, combine all the ingredients in a blender or food processor and blend until smooth. Set aside.

2. Combine all of the ingredients for pancakes in a food processor and blend until smooth.

3. Spray a skillet with nonstick cooking spray and heat over medium heat.

4. Ladle two spoonfuls of the mixture into the skillet and spread with spoon to make a thin circle. Cook until light brown on both sides (about 2 minutes).

5. Wrap pancake like a crepe, or lay flat.

6. Spoon a tablespoon of sauce over each pancake and serve.

Per serving: Calories 189; total fat 3 g; saturated fat 1 g; cholesterol 6 mg; sodium 378 mg; carbohydrates 25 g; dietary fiber 3 g; sugars 10 g; protein 16 g

Old Fashioned Eggs and Bacon
HMS, GS, SS

What can I say? It's a tradition!

MAKES 1 SERVING

2 eggs, preferably organic
2 slices nitrite-free turkey bacon

1. Spray a skillet with nonstick cooking spray and set it on medium heat. When it's hot, break the eggs into the pan and "fry" them to your desired doneness.

2. Cook the bacon in a separate pan or in the microwave.

Per serving: Calories 213; total fat 12.5 g; saturated fat 3 g; cholesterol 422 mg; sodium 542 mg; carbohydrates 1 g; dietary fiber 0 g; sugars 0 g; protein 25 g

Sweet Lemon Ricotta Pancakes with Blueberry Coulis

GS, SS

I had these at a hotel once and fell in love with them. This is my healthier version of that recipe.

MAKES 3 SERVINGS

For the coulis:

2 cups blueberries

2 tablespoons light agave syrup

2 tablespoon fresh lemon juice

For the pancakes:

1 cup fat-free ricotta cheese

1 cup skim milk

4 egg whites

1/4 cup Truvia

Zest and juice of 1 lemon

1 1/2 cups whole wheat flour

1 tablespoon baking powder

1. To make the coulis, combine the blueberries, agave syrup, and lemon juice in a food processor and pulse until the blueberries are crushed but not liquefied. Put in a small bowl and set aside.

2. In a food processor, add ricotta cheese, milk, egg whites, Truvia, lemon zest, and lemon juice until smooth.

3. Blend in the flour and baking powder.

4. Spray a griddle with nonstick cooking spray and heat it over medium heat. Ladle 2 tablespoons of batter onto the heated

griddle for each pancake. With spoon, smooth into a thin circle and cook until light brown on both sides, turning it once.

5. If you like, you can heat the coulis in a small pan while the pancakes cook, or simply spoon it on the cooked pancakes at room temperature.

Per serving: Calories 398; total fat 2 g; saturated fat 0 g; cholesterol 22 mg; sodium 673 mg; carbohydrates 77 g; dietary fiber 9 g; sugars 25 g; protein 24 g

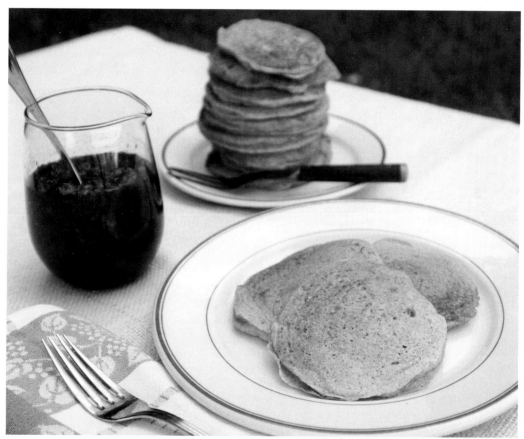

Good Morning Muffins

SS

MAKES 6 MUFFINS

¾ cup whole wheat flour
¾ cup oat bran cereal
½ teaspoon baking soda
1 teaspoon pumpkin pie spice
½ cup Truvia
½ teaspoon sea salt
½ cup 2 percent fat Greek yogurt
1 ripe banana, mashed
1 egg white and 1 whole egg, preferably organic, beaten together
2 tablespoons unsweetened applesauce
1 teaspoon vanilla extract
½ cup chopped walnuts
1 carrot, peeled and grated

1. Preheat the oven to 425°F.

2. Line the cups of a six-cup muffin tin with paper liners.

3. In one bowl, combine the flour, cereal, baking soda, pumpkin pie spice, Truvia, and salt.

4. In a second bowl, combine the yogurt, banana, eggs, applesauce, and vanilla.

5. With a mixing spoon, stir the wet ingredients into the dry.

6. Stir in the nuts and grated carrot.

7. Spoon the batter into the muffin cups and bake for 10 to 15 minutes, or until a toothpick inserted in the center of a muffin comes out clean.

Per serving: Calories 190; total fat 8 g; saturated fat 1 g; cholesterol 32 mg; sodium 290 mg; carbohydrates 27 g; dietary fiber 4 g; sugars 5.5 g; protein 8 g

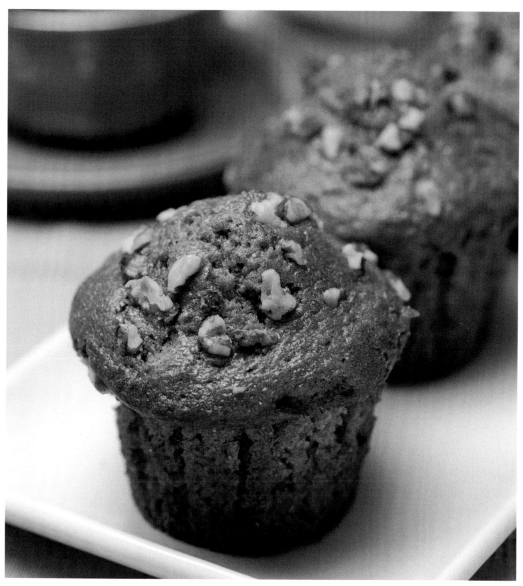

Lunch

Tarragon Chicken Salad

HMS, GS, SS

MAKES 1 SERVING

4 cups mixed salad greens
½ cup sliced fresh mushrooms
1 tablespoon sliced red onion
1 (4–6 ounce) grilled chicken breast, sliced into strips
1 ripe tomato, sliced
½ cucumber, sliced
1 tablespoon fresh lime juice
2 teaspoons extra-virgin olive oil
1 tablespoon chopped fresh tarragon
Sea salt to taste
Freshly ground pepper to taste

1. Combine mixed greens, mushrooms, onion, tomato, and cucumber in a bowl.

2. Blend lime juice, olive oil, and tarragon in food processor until smooth.

3. Pour the dressing over the salad and season with salt and pepper to taste.

Per serving: Calories 364; total fat 14 g; saturated fat 3 g; cholesterol 96 mg; sodium 313 mg; carbohydrates 219 g; dietary fiber 5 g; sugars 8 g; protein 41 g

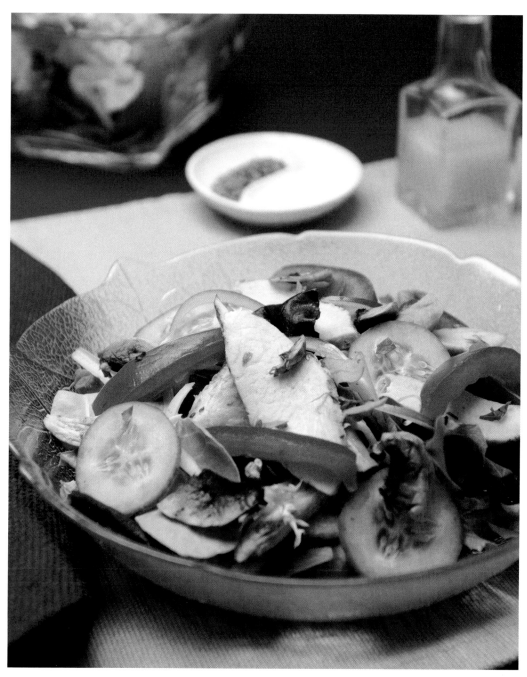

Grilled Chicken, Tomato, and Arugula Salad

MAKES 1 SERVING

4 cups arugula leaves
¼ cup coarsely chopped tomato
1 (4–6 ounce) grilled chicken breast, sliced

For the dressing:
1 garlic clove
2 teaspoons olive oil
1 tablespoon fresh lemon juice
½ teaspoon fresh or dried oregano

1. Place arugula on a plate. Sprinkle with chopped tomatoes, and layer with sliced chicken

2. Add all the ingredients for the dressing to a mini chopper and pulse until blended.

3. Pour the dressing over the salad mixture and toss.

Per serving: Calories 305; total fat 14 g; saturated fat 2.5 g; cholesterol 96 mg; sodium 109 mg; carbohydrates 7 g; dietary fiber 4 g; sugars 3 g; protein 38 g

Q & C Grilled Scallop Salad with Basil Vinaigrette

HMS, GS, SS

MAKES 1 SERVING

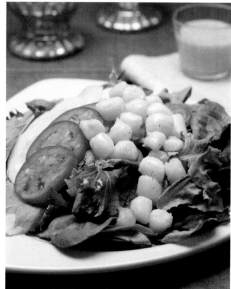

6 large raw sea scallops or
*   3 ounces bay scallops*
Sea salt and freshly ground pepper
*   to taste*
4 cups lettuce of your choice
1 cucumber, sliced
4 plum tomatoes, sliced
2 teaspoons extra-virgin olive oil
Juice of 1 lemon
3 basil leaves

1. Spray a grill pan with olive oil cooking spray and set over medium heat.

2. Sprinkle the scallops with the salt and pepper and grill them for about 3 minutes on each side, until firm. Remove from the heat and set aside.

3. Arrange the lettuce, cucumber, and tomatoes on a plate. When the scallops have cooled a bit, place them over the salad.

4. In a mini food processor, combine the olive oil, lemon juice, and basil leaves; pulse until blended. Pour over the salad, sprinkle with a bit more sea salt and pepper, and serve.

Per serving: Calories 305; total fat 11 g; saturated fat 2 g; cholesterol 28 mg; sodium 372 mg; carbohydrates 36 g; dietary fiber 10 g; sugars 17 g; protein 22 g

Grilled Shrimp and Cannellini Bean Salad

HMS, GS, SS

This dish is packed with protein and full of texture.

MAKES 1 SERVING

1½ tablespoons extra-virgin olive oil, divided
1 teaspoon chopped fresh garlic
Sea salt and freshly ground pepper to taste
6 large shrimp, cleaned and deveined
4 cups arugula
1 tablespoon sliced red onion
½ cup cooked cannellini beans (preferably organic), fresh or canned
1 tablespoon fresh lemon juice
1 tablespoon chopped parsley
2 teaspoons pine nuts

1. In a bowl, whisk 2 teaspoons of the olive oil with garlic and salt and pepper to taste. Add the shrimp and toss to coat well.

2. Generously spray a grill pan with nonstick cooking spray and set it over medium heat. When the pan is hot, grill the shrimp for 2 minutes on each side, just until pink and opaque. Don't overcook them or they will become rubbery. Remove from the pan and set aside.

3. In a large salad bowl, combine the arugula, onion, and cannellini beans, then add the shrimp.

4. In a mini food processor, blend the lemon juice, the remaining olive oil, and the parsley. Drizzle over the salad and toss to coat all the ingredients.

5. Sprinkle with the pine nuts and serve.

Per serving: Calories 359; total fat 19 g; saturated fat 2.5 g; cholesterol 64 mg; sodium 288 mg; carbohydrates 30 g; dietary fiber 8 g; sugars 3 g; protein 20.5 g

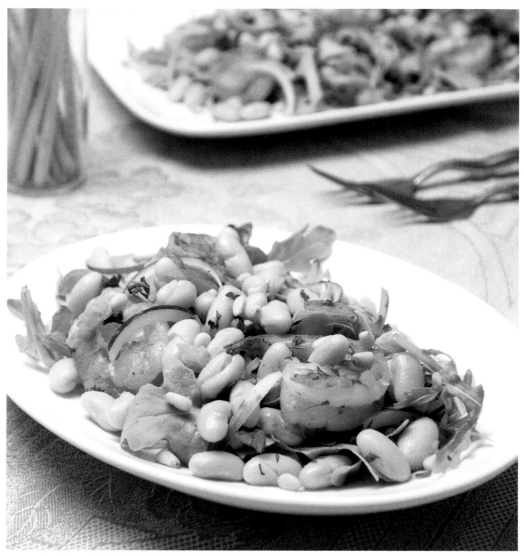

Sizzling Mini Pork Tacos with Peach Salsa
GS, SS

This is a fun dish to make on a Saturday night or when you just feel like eating something special. You can refrigerate the salsa in an airtight container for up to a week.

MAKES 2 SERVINGS

For the salsa:

3 ½ cups diced frozen or fresh peaches (about 2 ½ pounds)

¼ cup diced red onion

2 tablespoons finely chopped fresh cilantro

1 tablespoon minced seeded jalapeño pepper (optional)

2 teaspoons fresh lime juice

1 teaspoon fresh lemon juice

1 garlic clove, minced

1 teaspoon light agave syrup (if needed)*

For the tacos:

1 pound lean pork tenderloin, cut in thin strips

½ teaspoon ground cumin

½ teaspoon paprika

2 garlic cloves, chopped

Pinch of sea salt

6 mini whole wheat tortillas

1. Combine all the salsa ingredients and set aside.

2. In a bowl, toss the pork with the cumin, paprika, garlic, and salt.

3. Generously coat a grill pan with nonstick cooking spray and heat on medium. Add the pork and grill on both sides until cooked through.

4. Divide the pork filling among the tortillas and top with the salsa.

Per serving: Calories 683; total fat 14 g; saturated fat 5 g; cholesterol 143 mg; sodium 768 mg; carbohydrates 79 g; dietary fiber 13 g; sugars 28 g; protein 61 g

---

* If you are using ripe sweet fresh peaches you may not need the syrup, but if they are frozen and a little bitter, it might help the recipe.

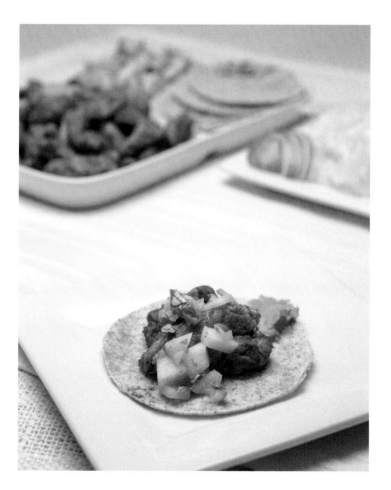

Creamy Chicken Salad

HMS, GS, SS

MAKES 1 SERVING

> 3 tablespoons plain low-fat yogurt
> 2 teaspoons Dijon mustard
> 1 teaspoon low-sodium soy sauce
> 1 teaspoon Truvia
> 1½ cups cubed cooked skinless, boneless chicken breast
> ¼ cup chopped celery
> 2 tablespoons chopped scallion
> 2 cups torn lettuce leaves of your choice
> Sea salt to taste

1. In a small bowl, combine the yogurt, mustard, soy sauce, and Truvia. Stir until blended.

2. In a large bowl, combine the chicken, celery, and scallion.

3. Pour the yogurt dressing over the chicken and mix well.

4. Arrange the lettuce on a plate, top with the chicken salad, sprinkle with sea salt, and serve.

Per serving: Calories 243; total fat 5 g; saturated fat 2 g; cholesterol 99 mg; sodium 771 mg; carbohydrates 9.5 g; dietary fiber 3 g; sugars 5 g; protein 39.5 g

Chopped Greek Chicken Salad

HMS, GS, SS

MAKES 2 SERVINGS

2 (4–6 ounce) uncooked skinless, boneless chicken breasts,
   pounded thin
1 bag mixed lettuce greens (or as much as you want)
1 cucumber, chopped
1 tomato, cut in small cubes
1 red onion, peeled and chopped
8 black olives, chopped
1½ tablespoons extra-virgin olive oil
2 tablespoons fresh lemon juice
1 teaspoon dried oregano
Freshly ground pepper to taste
1 tablespoon crumbled feta cheese

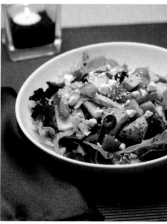

1. Spray a grill pan with nonstick cooking spray and set it over medium heat.

2. Grill the chicken breasts about 3 minutes on each side or until done. Set aside to cool.

3. Combine the lettuce, chopped cucumber, tomato, onion, and olives in a salad bowl.

4. Chop the cooled chicken and add it to the bowl.

5. Whisk together the olive oil and lemon juice and pour the dressing over the salad. Sprinkle with the oregano and pepper to taste. Top with the cheese.

Per serving: Calories 328; total fat 16 g; saturated fat 3 g; cholesterol 76 mg; sodium 332 mg; carbohydrates 19 g; dietary fiber 5 g; sugars 7.5 g; protein 28.5 g

Mexican Soup

HMS, GS, SS

Freeze any leftovers in individual portion containers to have on hand for a quick lunch when you're in a hurry.

MAKES ABOUT 4 CUPS

2 (4–6 ounce) skinless, boneless chicken breasts, sliced in thin strips
2 garlic cloves, minced
1 cup chopped celery
1 cup chopped green pepper
¼ cup chopped tomato
1 cup chopped carrots
1 cup chopped onion
½ teaspoon ground cumin
½ teaspoon dried oregano
4 cups low-sodium chicken broth
Sea salt to taste
1 tablespoon chopped cilantro

1. Spray a large nonstick pot or Dutch oven with nonstick cooking spray.

2. Set over medium heat and add the chicken. Sauté for about 5 minutes or until cooked through.

3. Add all the vegetables and stir to combine. Add the cumin and oregano and cook until the vegetables begin to soften. Add the chicken broth, reduce the heat to low, stir, and continue to cook for about 20 minutes, stirring frequently.

4. Add sea salt to taste. Sprinkle with the cilantro and serve.

Per cup: Calories 149; total fat 3 g; saturated fat 1 g; cholesterol 36 mg; sodium 232 mg; carbohydrates 13 g; dietary fiber 3 g; sugars 5 g; protein 18 g

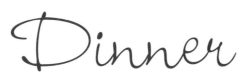

Dinner

Shrimp Taco Lettuce Wraps

HMS, GS, SS

In this recipe tender Boston lettuce leaves substitute for traditional taco shells.

MAKES 1 SERVING

> 1 tablespoon canola oil
> 3–4 ounces large raw shrimp, peeled, deveined, and chopped
> 1 teaspoon chopped garlic
> ¼ cup bean sprouts
> 4 large Boston lettuce leaves
> 1 small tomato, chopped
> 1 teaspoon chopped cilantro
> ½ lime
> Sea salt and freshly ground pepper to taste

1. Heat the oil in a medium skillet.

2. Add the shrimp, garlic, and beans sprouts. Sauté, stirring, until the shrimp are just pink.

3. Lay the lettuce leaves on a platter or individual plates and spoon the shrimp mixture over them.

4. Add the chopped tomato, sprinkle with cilantro, drizzle with lime juice, and season with salt and pepper.

Per serving: Calories 232; total fat 12 g; saturated fat 1 g; cholesterol 129 mg; sodium 333 mg; carbohydrates 13 g; dietary fiber 4 g; sugars 5 g; protein 20 g

Super-Clean Shrimp and Broccoli

HMS, GS, SS

MAKES 2 SERVINGS

¼ cup fat-free low-sodium chicken broth
2 tablespoons low-sodium soy sauce
1 tablespoon canola oil, divided
1 tablespoon peeled, minced fresh ginger
3 garlic cloves, chopped
12 peeled and deveined uncooked extra-large shrimp
2 cups small broccoli florets
2 tablespoons chopped scallions

1. In a small bowl, whisk together the chicken broth and soy sauce.

2. Heat 2 teaspoons of the canola oil in a large nonstick skillet over medium-high heat.

3. Add the ginger and garlic. Stir-fry 30 seconds.

4. Add the shrimp and stir-fry 3 minutes longer, or until the shrimp is slightly pink. Remove the shrimp mixture from the pan and set aside.

5. Add the remaining 1 teaspoon of canola oil to the pan. Add the broccoli and scallions and stir-fry 2 minutes, or until the broccoli is crisp-tender.

6. Return the shrimp mixture to the pan, add the broth mixture, and cook, stirring constantly, for 1 minute.

Per serving: Calories 388; total fat 10 g; saturated fat 1 g; cholesterol 577.5 mg; sodium 1241 mg; carbohydrates 16 g; dietary fiber 3 g; sugars 3 g; protein 68 g

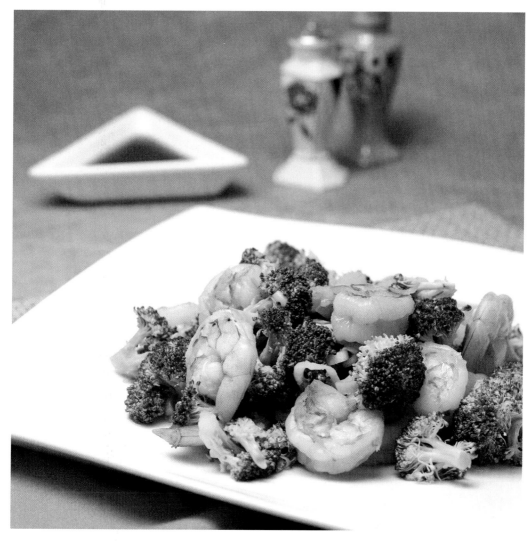

Chicken Stir-Fry with Cashews

GS, SS

MAKES 1 SERVING

1 tablespoon canola oil

1 (4–6 ounce) skinless, boneless chicken breast, pounded thin and
  sliced

3 garlic cloves

1 medium red pepper, cored, seeded, and sliced

1 teaspoon peeled and chopped fresh ginger

2 cups snow peas

2 tablespoons Bragg's Liquid Aminos

1 tablespoon coarsely chopped unsalted cashews

1. Heat the oil in a wok or skillet. Add the chicken, garlic, and pepper; stir-fry until the chicken is almost cooked through.

2. Add the ginger and snow peas and stir-fry for a minute or two until the peas are bright green.

3. Add the Bragg's and cashews and toss once or twice. Remove from the heat and serve.

Per serving: Calories 529; total fat 24 g; saturated fat 3 g; cholesterol 145 mg; sodium 1,601 mg; carbohydrates 24 g; dietary fiber 6 g; sugars 11 g; protein 58 g

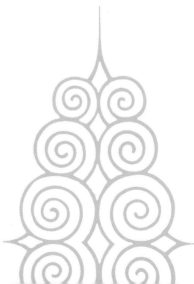

Rosemary Dijon Chicken Breast over Steamed Spinach

HMS, GS, SS

MAKES 1 SERVING

1 (4–6 ounce) skinless, boneless chicken breast, pounded thin
Salt to taste
½ teaspoon freshly ground black pepper
1 tablespoon extra-virgin olive oil
3 tablespoons chopped shallot
¼ cup fat-free, low-sodium chicken broth
¼ cup water
1 sprig rosemary
2 teaspoons Dijon mustard
2 cups baby spinach leaves

1. Sprinkle the chicken with salt and pepper.

2. Heat the oil in a large skillet over medium-high heat, add the chicken, and sauté for 3 minutes on each side, or until cooked through.

3. Transfer the chicken to a serving platter, and add the shallot to the pan. Sauté for 2 minutes, then stir in the chicken broth and water, add the rosemary sprig, and bring to a boil. Cook for 2 minutes, then remove from the heat, discard the rosemary, and stir in the mustard.

4. Spread the spinach on a plate, top with the chicken, and spoon the sauce over all. Let sit for a minute or two until the spinach wilts.

Per serving: Calories 392; total fat 14 g; saturated fat 3 g; cholesterol 145 mg; sodium 890 mg; carbohydrates 11 g; dietary fiber 3 g; sugars 1 g; protein 53 g

Chicken Marsala

HMS, GS, SS

MAKES 1 SERVING

> 1 cup sliced mushrooms
> 2 tablespoons low-sodium chicken broth
> 1 (4–6 ounce) skinless, boneless chicken breast, pounded thin
> 1 teaspoon cornstarch
> ¼ cup Marsala or dry white wine

1. Spray a nonstick skillet generously with nonstick cooking spray and set it over medium heat. Add the mushrooms and cook, stirring, until softened. Remove from the pan and set aside.

2. Add the chicken broth to the pan and heat to a simmer. (You may have to spray pan again.)

3. Add the chicken breasts and cook for 3 minutes on each side. Remove from the pan and set aside.

4. Mix the cornstarch and wine in a small bowl, then add to skillet and stir until thickened.

5. Return the chicken and mushrooms to the pan until just heated through.

Per serving: Calories 288; total fat 4 g; saturated fat 1 g; cholesterol 91 mg; sodium 558.5 mg; carbohydrates 14 g; dietary fiber 1 g; sugars 2 g; protein 34 g

Olive Oil Herb-Roasted Flank Steak

HMS, GS, SS

MAKES 4 SERVINGS

2 tablespoons extra-virgin olive oil
1 teaspoon chopped fresh thyme
1 teaspoon chopped fresh parsley
1 teaspoon chopped fresh rosemary
3 garlic cloves, minced
1 teaspoon sea salt
1½ pounds flank steak, trimmed of visible fat

1. In a large bowl, combine the olive oil, herbs, garlic, and sea salt. Mix well.

2. Score the surface of the steak so that the marinade can permeate the meat. Add it to the bowl, turning to coat it well. Cover and refrigerate for at least 30 minutes and no more than 4 hours.

3. Meanwhile, preheat the oven to 400°F.

4. Transfer the steak and its juices to a large ovenproof pan and roast for about 40 minutes or until cooked to your liking.

Per serving: Calories 306; total fat 16 g; saturated fat 6 g; cholesterol 69 mg; sodium 204 mg; carbohydrates 1 g; dietary fiber 0 g; sugars 0 g; protein 37 g

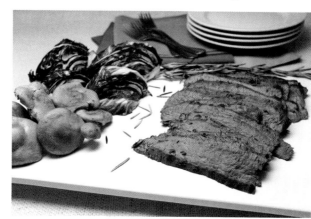

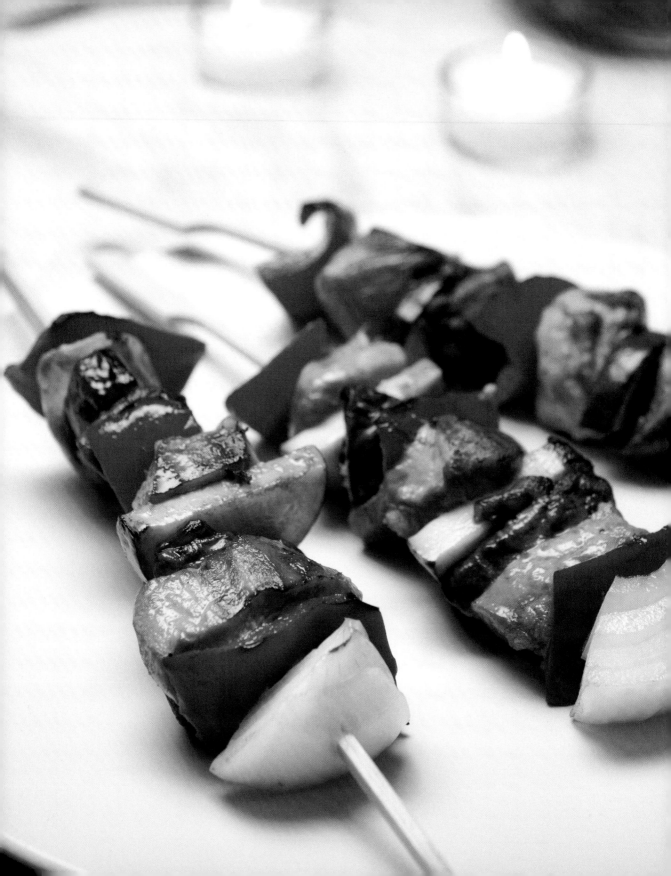

Q & C Grilled Chicken Kebabs

HMS, GS, SS

MAKES 1 SERVING

2 tablespoons low-sodium soy sauce
2 garlic cloves, chopped
1 tablespoon sesame oil
1 (4–6 ounce) skinless, boneless chicken breast, cubed
1 small zucchini, cubed
1½ cups quartered large mushrooms
1 cup red bell pepper squares
1 large onion, cut in squares

1. In a large bowl, combine the soy sauce, garlic, and sesame oil. Mix well.

2. Add the chicken and vegetables and marinate in the refrigerator for at least 1 hour.

3. Remove the chicken and vegetables from the bowl. Reserve the marinade.

4. Thread the marinated ingredients onto skewers, alternating chicken and vegetables. If you are using wooden skewers, be sure to soak them in water for at least 10 minutes before using.

5. Heat a grill or grill pan to medium.

6. Brush the kebabs with the reserved marinade and grill for about 5 minutes on each side, or until done.

Per serving: Calories 393; total fat 10 g; saturated fat 2 g; cholesterol 91 mg; sodium 564 mg; carbohydrates 37 g; dietary fiber 10 g; sugars 22 g; protein 42 g

Beef and Scallop Kebabs with Grilled Vegetables

HMS, GS, SS

MAKES 2 SERVINGS

½ cup Bragg's Liquid Aminos, divided
1 tablespoon fresh lemon juice
2 garlic cloves, finely chopped
3 ounces lean beef, cubed
3 ounces sea scallops
½ teaspoon garlic powder
1 zucchini, cubed
8 mushrooms, cut in quarters
1 medium onion, cut in chunks
12 cherry or grape tomatoes
1 tablespoon canola oil

1. Combine ¼ cup of the Bragg's, the lemon juice, and the garlic in a bowl large enough to hold the meat.

2. Pat the beef dry, add it to the marinade, turn to coat well, and refrigerate for at least 30 minutes.

3. When you are ready to cook, put the scallops in a bowl and sprinkle with the remaining Bragg's and the garlic powder.

4. Brush the vegetables with the canola oil.

5. Heat the grill. While it is heating, skewer the beef and half the vegetables on one set of skewers and the scallops and remaining vegetables on another set. If you are using wooden skewers, be sure to soak them in water for at least 10 minutes before using.

6. Put the beef skewers on the grill first, as they will take longer to cook. When the beef is almost done, add the scallop skewers and grill just until the scallops are opaque. If you overcook them, they will become rubbery.

7. Remove from the heat and serve.

Per serving: Calories 249; total fat 10 g; saturated fat 2 g; cholesterol 42 mg; sodium 778 mg; carbohydrates 20 g; dietary fiber 5 g; sugars 11 g; protein 24 g

Poached Halibut with Capers

HMS, GS, SS

This is a great, light dinner to serve with a green salad.

MAKES 1 SERVING

1 tablespoon olive oil
2 teaspoons fresh lemon juice
1 shallot, chopped
1 (4–6 ounce) halibut fillet
2 teaspoons capers
Freshly ground pepper to taste

1. Whisk the oil, lemon juice, and shallot together until emulsified. Set aside.

2. Fill a wide, shallow saucepan with water and bring to a boil.

3. Reduce the heat to a simmer, add the halibut, and poach until opaque and cooked through.

4. Transfer to a serving platter, pour the lemon dressing over the fish, sprinkle with the capers and fresh pepper, and serve.

Per serving: Calories 288; total fat 16 g; saturated fat 2 g; cholesterol 83 mg; sodium 397 mg; carbohydrates 2.5 g; dietary fiber 0 g; sugars 1 g; protein 32 g

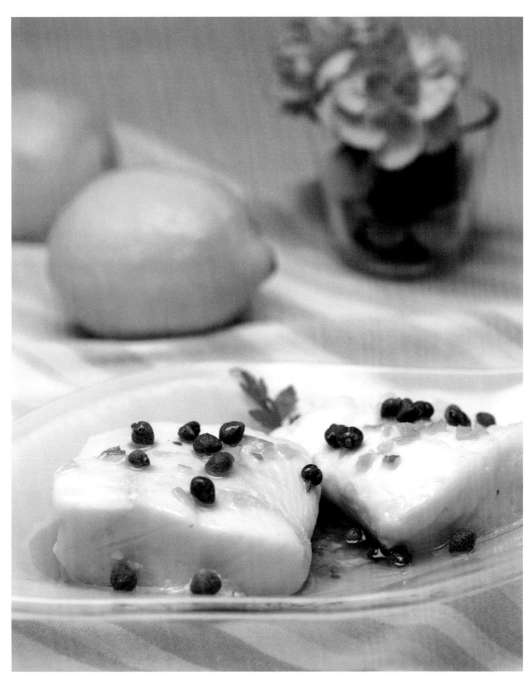

Salmon with Snow Peas and Fresh Dill

HMS, GS, SS

MAKES 1 SERVING

> *1 (4–6 ounce) salmon fillet*
> *1 tablespoon extra-virgin olive oil*
> *2 cups snow peas, steamed*
> *1 tablespoon chopped fresh dill*
> *2 tablespoons chopped chives*
> *Sea salt to taste*
> *Juice of ½ lemon*

1. Rub the salmon with the olive oil.

2. Spray a skillet with nonstick cooking spray and set it over medium heat. Add the salmon and cook until firm on both sides.

3. Arrange the steamed snow peas on a plate, top with the salmon, and sprinkle with the dill, chives, and sea salt.

4. Squeeze the lemon over all, and serve.

Per serving: Calories 378; total fat 15 g; saturated fat 2 g; cholesterol 62 mg; sodium 261 mg; carbohydrates 30 g; dietary fiber 12.5 g; sugars 15 g; protein 35 g

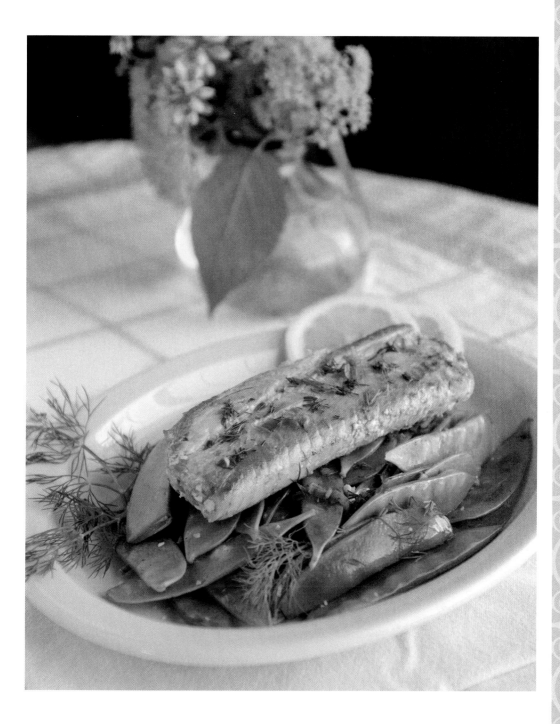

Garlic Lime Chicken
on a Bed of Steamed Spinach

HMS, GS, SS

MAKES 2 SERVINGS

¹⁄₄ cup fresh lime juice
2 garlic cloves, chopped
¹⁄₂ teaspoon mustard powder
2 skinless, boneless chicken breasts
1 (10-ounce) bag baby spinach leaves or 1 box frozen spinach

1. In a bowl, whisk together the lime, garlic, and mustard powder. Add the chicken, turning to coat it well, and marinate in the refrigerator for 30 minutes. You can do this up to 4 hours ahead of time.

2. When you're ready to cook, heat the oven to 350°F.

3. Place the chicken in an ovenproof pan and pour the marinade over it. Bake for 20 minutes or until cooked through.

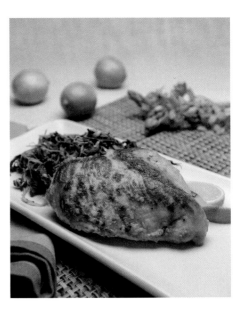

4. While chicken is cooking, steam the fresh spinach or cook the frozen according to package directions.

5. To serve, arrange the chicken over the spinach.

Per serving: Calories 177; total fat 3 g; saturated fat 1 g; cholesterol 73 mg; sodium 241 mg; carbohydrates 9 g; dietary fiber 4 g; sugars 1 g; protein 28 g

Balsamic Chicken
with Steamed Brussels Sprouts

HMS, GS, SS

MAKES 1 SERVING

2 garlic cloves, minced
2 tablespoons olive oil
¼ cup balsamic vinegar
Sea salt and freshly ground pepper to taste
2 (4–6 ounce) skinless, boneless chicken breasts, pounded thin
2 cups brussels sprouts
Juice of ½ lemon

1. In a medium bowl, whisk together the garlic, oil, vinegar, salt, and pepper. Add the chicken, turning to coat it on all sides, and marinate in the refrigerator for at least 30 minutes and no longer than 4 hours.

2. When ready to cook, heat the oven to 350°F.

3. Spray a small ovenproof pan with nonstick cooking spray.

4. Drain the chicken from the marinade, transfer it to the pan, and bake about 10 minutes or until cooked through.

5. While the chicken is baking, steam the brussels sprouts.

6. When ready to serve, transfer the chicken and sprouts to a serving platter and squeeze the lemon juice over the sprouts.

Per serving: Calories 336; total fat 9 g; saturated fat 1 g; cholesterol 109 mg; sodium 266 mg; carbohydrates 25 g; dietary fiber 9 g; sugars 6.5 g; protein 43 g

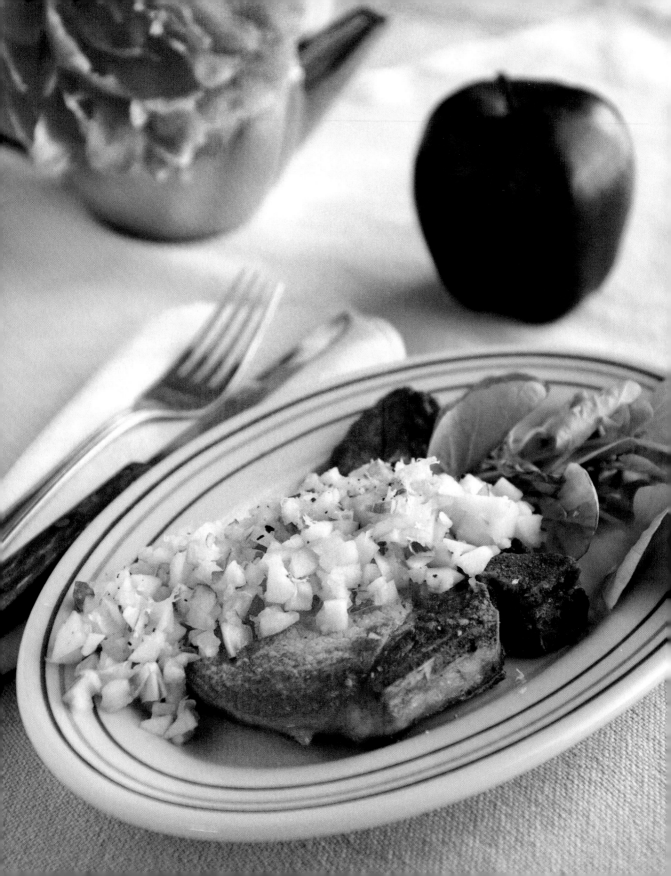

Grilled Pork Chops
with Red Onion Apple Relish

HMS, GS, SS

I like to serve these chops with a green salad on the side.

MAKES 2 SERVINGS

2 bone-in lean pork chops
Sea salt and freshly ground pepper to taste
½ Red Delicious apple, peeled, cored, and chopped
¼ cup chopped red onion
1 tablespoon fresh lemon juice
1 teaspoon Truvia

1. Spray a grill or grill pan with nonstick cooking spray and heat.

2. Season the pork chops with salt and pepper.

3. Grill the chops, turning them once, for about 10 minutes or until cooked through. Remove from the heat and set aside.

4. In a saucepan, combine the apple, onion, lemon juice, and Truvia. Heat until the apples soften.

5. Spoon the relish over the chops and serve.

Per serving: Calories 186; total fat 6 g; saturated fat 2 g; cholesterol 63.5 mg; sodium 166.5 mg; carbohydrates 9 g; dietary fiber 1 g; sugars 5.5 g; protein 25 g

Sautéed Shrimp with Arugula and Tomatoes

HMS, GS, SS

MAKES 2 SERVINGS

1 ½ tablespoons olive oil

2 garlic cloves, chopped

1 cup grape tomatoes

12 large uncooked shrimp, peeled and deveined

1 bunch arugula, washed and stemmed

1 tablespoon fresh lemon juice

Sea salt and freshly ground pepper to taste

1. In a large skillet, heat the oil over medium heat. Add the garlic and sauté, being careful not to let it burn.

2. When the garlic is soft, add the tomatoes and toss once or twice.

3. Add the shrimp and cook just until pink.

4. Add the arugula and toss until the greens are wilted.

5. Sprinkle with lemon juice and season with salt and pepper.

Per serving: Calories 340; total fat 13 g; saturated fat 2 g; cholesterol 345 mg; sodium 439 mg; carbohydrates 8 g; dietary fiber 1 g; sugars 3 g; protein 47 g

Sides

Grilled Vegetable Plate with Balsamic Drizzle

HMS, GS, SS

This could also be a vegetarian lunch or dinner for two.

MAKES 2 SERVINGS

2 zucchini, sliced on the diagonal
2 summer squash, sliced on the diagonal
1 large red bell pepper, cored, seeded, and sliced
1 cup halved yellow and red grape tomatoes
1 medium onion, sliced
2 tablespoons extra-virgin olive oil
2 tablespoons balsamic vinegar
Sea salt and freshly ground pepper to taste

1. Spray a grill or grill pan with nonstick cooking spray and set over medium heat.

2. Brush the vegetables with the oil and grill until tender, turning them once.

3. Transfer the grilled vegetables to a serving platter and drizzle with the vinegar. Season with salt and pepper to taste.

Per serving: Calories 189; total fat 6 g; saturated fat 1 g; cholesterol 0 mg; sodium 138 mg; carbohydrates 30 g; dietary fiber 8 g; sugars 21 g; protein 7 g

Steamed Broccoli Rabe with Lemon

HMS, GS, SS

MAKES 2 SERVINGS

1 bunch broccoli rabe, stems trimmed
2 teaspoons olive oil
Juice of ½ lemon
Red pepper flakes to taste

1. Steam the broccoli rabe until bright green and tender.

2. Transfer to a platter, drizzle with the olive oil and lemon juice, and sprinkle with red pepper flakes.

Per serving: Calories 66; total fat 5 g; saturated fat 1 g; cholesterol 6 mg; sodium 32 mg; carbohydrates 6 g; dietary fiber 4 g; sugars 1 g; protein 3 g

Steamed Spinach with Lemon

HMS

MAKES 2 SERVINGS

2 cups coarsely chopped spinach
1 teaspoon olive oil
Juice of ½ lemon
Sea salt to taste

Place the spinach into a steamer on top of boiling water. Cover and steam until the spinach is bright green but slightly wilted. Transfer to a platter; drizzle with olive oil, lemon juice, and salt to taste.

Per serving: Calories 32; total fat 2 g; saturated fat 0 g; cholesterol 0 mg; sodium 122 mg; carbohydrates 4 g; dietary fiber 2 g; sugars 1 g; protein 1 g

Q & C Lemon Agave Collards

GS, SS

MAKES 3 SERVINGS

> 1 tablespoon fresh lemon juice
> 1 teaspoon agave syrup
> 2 tablespoons extra-virgin olive oil
> 3 garlic cloves, chopped
> 1½ pounds collard greens, well washed and coarsely chopped
> 1 teaspoon sea salt

1. In a small bowl, combine the lemon juice and agave syrup.

2. In a nonstick skillet, heat the olive oil and add the garlic, stirring until it is translucent but not browned.

3. Add the collards and toss with the garlic until they begin to wilt. When they become very dark green, remove from the heat and transfer to a serving dish.

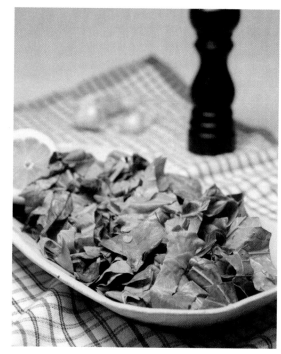

4. Toss with sea salt and drizzle with the lemon agave mixture.

Per serving: Calories 138; total fat 8 g; saturated fat 1 g; cholesterol 16 mg; sodium 566 mg; carbohydrates 16 g; dietary fiber 8 g; sugars 2 g; protein 6 g

Crispy Kale with Maple-Glazed Shallots

GS, SS

MAKES 1 SERVING

1 teaspoon fresh lemon juice
2 teaspoons maple syrup
2 teaspoons olive oil
4 small shallots, peeled and sliced crosswise
1 bunch fresh kale, washed thoroughly and coarsely chopped
Sea salt to taste

1. In a small bowl, combine the lemon juice and maple syrup.

2. In a nonstick skillet, heat the olive oil; add the shallots and cook, stirring, until translucent.

3. Add the kale and toss with the shallots until it begins to wilt. When the kale becomes very dark green, transfer it to a serving bowl, toss with the sea salt, and drizzle with the lemon-and-maple mixture.

Per serving: Calories 173; total fat 8 g; saturated fat 1 g; cholesterol 0 mg; sodium 257 mg; carbohydrates 26 g; dietary fiber 4 g; sugars 12 g; protein 5 g

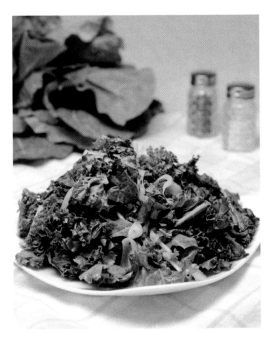

Brown Rice Delight

SS

MAKES 4 SERVINGS

1 cup uncooked brown rice
$\frac{1}{2}$ cup low-sodium vegetable
  stock
1 tablespoon olive oil
1 red onion, chopped
1 red bell pepper, cored,
  seeded, and chopped
1 carrot, chopped
1 celery stalk, chopped
$\frac{1}{2}$ cup chopped mushrooms
$\frac{1}{2}$ cup cleaned, trimmed, and
  chopped leeks
$\frac{1}{4}$ cup equal parts chopped
  parsley, basil, and thyme
Dash of Bragg's Liquid Aminos

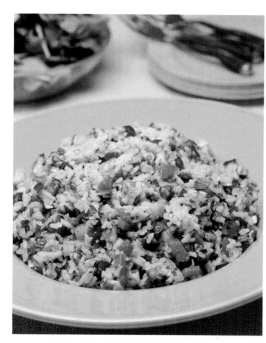

1. Cook the brown rice
   according to package instructions, using the vegetable stock
   as part of the cooking liquid.

2. While the rice is cooking, heat the oil in a skillet and sauté
   the vegetables until tender but still somewhat crisp.

3. When the rice is cooked, toss it with the vegetables, add the
   herbs, sprinkle with the Bragg's, and serve.

Per serving: Calories 236; total fat 4 g; saturated fat 1 g; cholesterol
0 mg; sodium 103 mg; carbohydrates 45 g; dietary fiber 4 g; sugars
5 g; protein 5 g

Snacks

Except for a few, the following are not complete recipes but rather suggestions for snack choices that will add more variety to all stages of the Quick & Clean Diet.

Strawberry Greek Yogurt Parfait

HMS

I'm calling this a snack, but I also eat it for breakfast.

MAKES 1 SERVING

½ cup 2 percent fat Greek yogurt
2 teaspoons no-sugar-added strawberry jam
1 teaspoon sliced almonds

Layer all the ingredients in a parfait glass and enjoy.

Per serving: Calories 95; total fat 3 g; saturated fat 2 g; cholesterol 7.5 mg; sodium 32.5 mg; carbohydrates 8 g; dietary fiber 0 g; sugars 5 g; protein 10.5 g

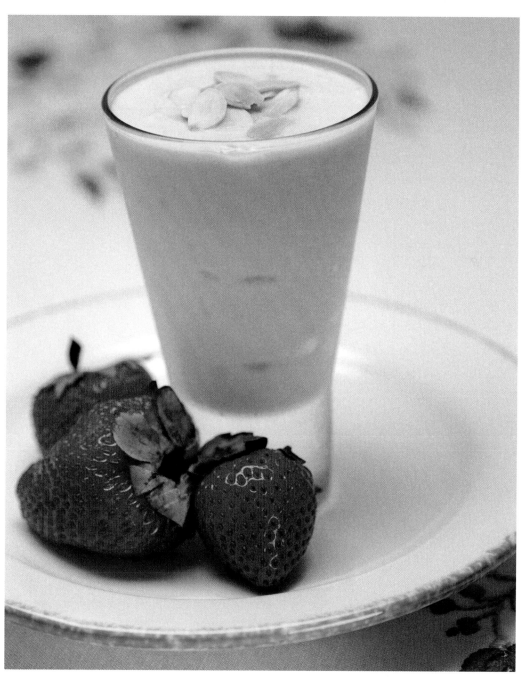

Ranch Dip

This dip goes well with raw vegetables and even works as a salad dressing. It keeps for several days in the refrigerator covered airtight.

MAKES ABOUT 12 SERVINGS

¾ cup nonfat or 2 percent fat Greek yogurt

⅓ cup Spectrum light canola mayo

1 teaspoon Worcestershire sauce

1 teaspoon garlic powder

1 teaspoon onion powder

1 teaspoon sea salt

1 tablespoon chopped flat-leaf parsley

1 tablespoon chopped chives

1 teaspoon white balsamic vinegar

1 cup 1 percent fat buttermilk

1. In a medium-size bowl, whisk together the yogurt, mayo, Worcestershire sauce, garlic powder, onion powder, salt, parsley, and chives.

2. Add the balsamic vinegar and buttermilk, and stir to emulsify.

3. Cover and refrigerate for an hour before serving.

Per serving: Calories 41; total fat 2 g; saturated fat 1 g; cholesterol 3 mg; sodium 204 mg; carbohydrates 3 g; dietary fiber 0 g; sugars 2 g; protein 2 g

Creamy Strawberry Cottage Cheese with Almonds

HMS

MAKES 1 SERVING

½ cup 2 percent fat cottage cheese
1 teaspoon no-sugar-added strawberry jam
1 teaspoon sliced almonds

Place cottage cheese in a small bowl. Spoon strawberry jam on top and sprinkle with almonds.

Per serving: Calories 113; total fat 4 g; saturated fat 1 g; cholesterol 11 mg; sodium 374 mg; carbohydrates 6 g; dietary fiber 0 g; sugars 4 g; protein 14 g

More snacks for all stages:

- ½ avocado and grape tomato halves drizzled with balsamic vinegar

- 4 steamed shrimp

- 1 apple, sliced, with 2 teaspoons almond butter

- ½ cup 2 percent fat cottage cheese with blueberries

- ½ cup mixed berries

- 1 cup 2 percent fat Greek yogurt with 1 packet Truvia and maple extract

- 1 pink grapefruit

Desserts

Caramelized Cinnamon Maple Bananas with Coconut Milk Ice Cream and Rum Sauce

SS

MAKES 1 SERVING

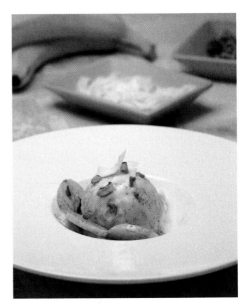

1 teaspoon ground cinnamon

1 tablespoon maple flakes (available in health food stores)

2 tablespoons rum extract

1 ripe banana, sliced

½ cup coconut milk ice cream (available in health food stores)

1 teaspoon chopped pecans (optional)

1. In a small bowl, combine the cinnamon, maple flakes, and rum extract. Mix until the maple flakes dissolve.

2. Add the banana and toss.

3. Scoop the ice cream into a bowl, add the sauce, and sprinkle with the nuts if desired.

Per serving: Calories 351; total fat 8 g; saturated fat 6.5 g; cholesterol 0 mg; sodium 17 mg; carbohydrates 51 g; dietary fiber 4 g; sugars 30 g; protein 2 g

Balsamic Strawberries with Basil Ribbons

SS

MAKES 2 SERVINGS

10 strawberries, hulled and sliced thin
1 tablespoon dark agave syrup
2 teaspoons balsamic vinegar
3 basil leaves, sliced very thin*

1. Pile the strawberries on a lovely plate.

2. In a small bowl, mix the agave syrup with the balsamic vinegar. Pour over the strawberries, and sprinkle with the basil.

Per serving: Calories 48; total fat 0 g; saturated fat 0 g; cholesterol 0 mg; sodium 2 mg; carbohydrates 12 g; dietary fiber 1 g; sugars 9 g; protein 0 g

---

* Stack the leaves, roll them up, and slice with your sharpest knife.

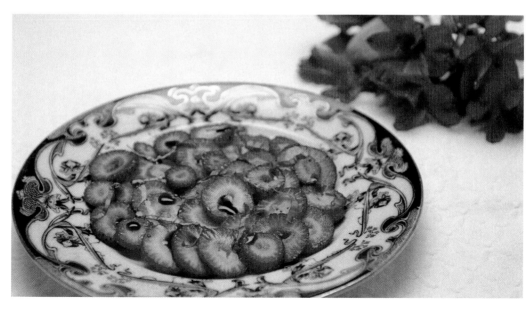

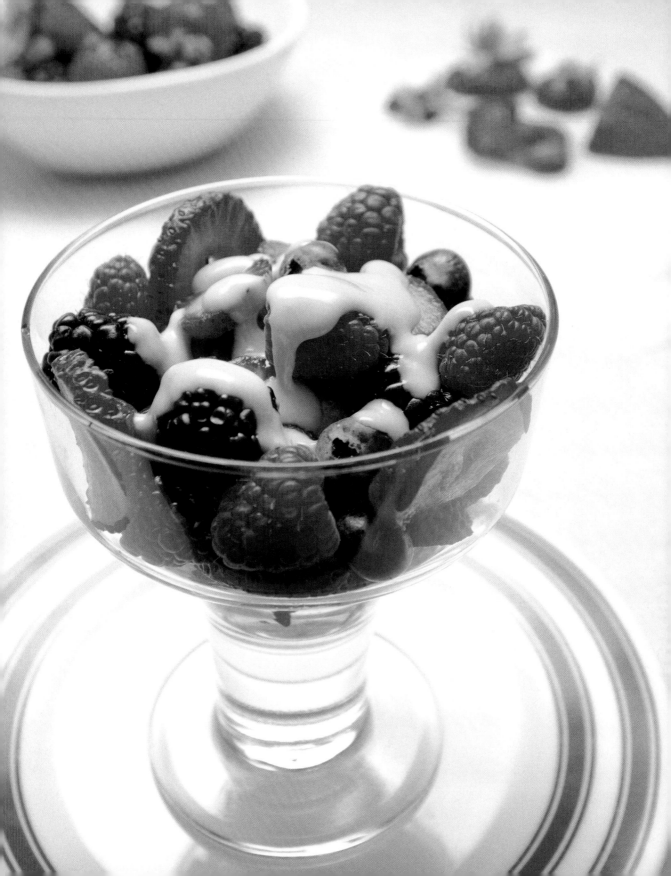

Mixed Berries with Vanilla Bean Cream

SS

MAKES 2 SERVINGS

> 2 tablespoons vanilla-flavored nonfat Greek yogurt
> 1½ teaspoons dark agave syrup, divided
> 1 teaspoon vanilla extract
> 5 strawberries, hulled and sliced
> 15 blueberries
> 5 raspberries
> 5 blackberries

1. In a small bowl, stir the yogurt with 1 teaspoon of the agave syrup and the vanilla until creamy.

2. Place the berries in a bowl, top with the cream, drizzle with the remaining ½ teaspoon of agave, and serve.

Per serving: Calories 49; total fat 0 g; saturated fat 0 g; cholesterol 0 mg; sodium 7.5 mg; carbohydrates 9.5 g; dietary fiber 2 g; sugars 7 g; protein 2 g

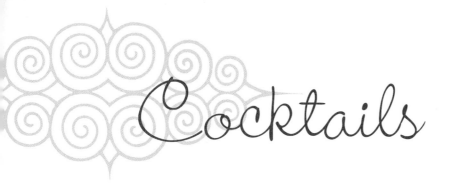

Cocktails

These are for the Stability Stage only!

A good drink means a lot to me. If you make a clean drink using fresh ingredients and the best liquor, it will not only taste great, but also be better for you. I prefer drinks on the rocks because the water content is higher, which is better for you, and you don't finish your drink as fast. All recipes make two drinks.

Q & C Classic Margarita on the Rocks!
SS

Skip the salt on the rim. You don't need that added sodium.

½ cup clear tequila
¾ cup fresh lime juice
2 teaspoons agave syrup
2 lime wedges, for garnish

1. Pour the tequila, lime juice, and agave into a shaker and shake until frothy.

2. Fill two glasses with ice and pour in the margarita mixture.

3. Garnish with the lime wedges and serve.

Per serving: Calories 166; total fat 0 g; saturated fat 0 g; cholesterol 0 mg; sodium 2 mg; carbohydrates 12 g; dietary fiber 0 g; sugars 5 g; protein 0 g

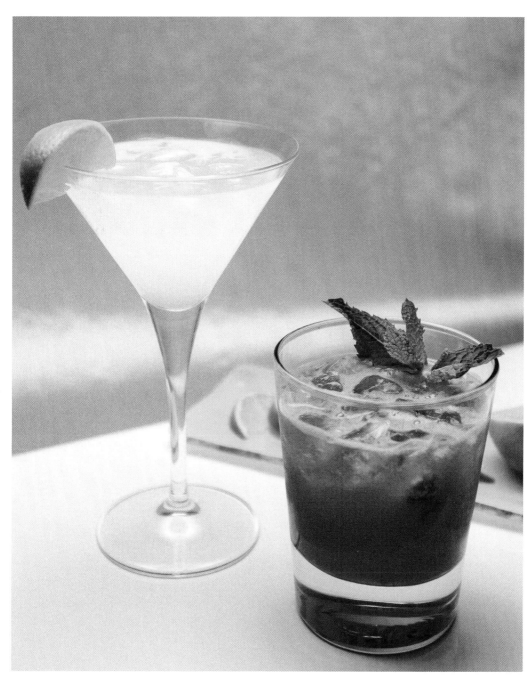

Q & C Pineapple Margarita on the Rocks

SS

½ cup clear tequila
6 tablespoons fresh lime juice
½ cup fresh or unsweetened pineapple juice
1½ teaspoons agave syrup
Crushed ice
2 lime slices, for garnish

1. Place all ingredients except the lime slices in a shaker and shake vigorously.

2. Pour into your favorite glasses and garnish with the lime slices.

Per serving: Calories 184; total fat 0 g; saturated fat 0 g; cholesterol 0 mg; sodium 2 mg; carbohydrates 15 g; dietary fiber 0 g; sugars 10 g; protein 0 g

Watermelon Gin Punch

SS

> ½ *cup good gin*
> *1 cup seeded and cubed watermelon*
> ¼ *cup fresh lime juice*
> *2 tablespoons agave syrup*
> *6 fresh mint leaves*

1. Combine the gin, watermelon, lime juice, and agave in a blender.

2. Put 3 mint leaves in the bottom of each glass and muddle with the back of a wooden spoon to release their flavor.

3. Add ice to the glasses and fill with the watermelon mixture.

Per serving: Calories 204; total fat 0 g; saturated fat 0 g; cholesterol 0 mg; sodium 2 mg; carbohydrates 20 g; dietary fiber 0 g; sugars 15 g; protein 1 g

Acknowledgments

There are so many! First, to the Blessed Mother, thank you for your love and guidance. May I be a source of strength to all women.

To my husband, for trying all my recipes and telling me the truth about them. To Laura Dail for her guidance and feedback.

To my friends at skirt! Books, especially Mary Norris—the best editor a writer can ask for. You are a true gem! There should be more in the business like you. To Ellen, Sheryl, Joanna, Casey, and Diana, thank you for your patience and fine work.

To Raphael B. for my amazing cover photo. Julie P. for your brilliant makeup and friendship.

My friends Linda P., Sherrie K., Fred M., and Byron H., for sampling, listening, and suggesting. I couldn't have done it without you.

XXOO,
D.A.

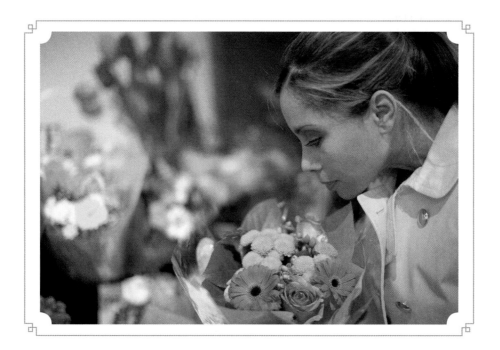

Index

Photo Credits

Photo © Julie Bidwell pages 2, 5, 7, 12, 18, 20, 22, 28, 33, 34, 36, 37, 40, 41, 42, 43, 44, 46, 47, 50, 51, 52, 55, 62, 66, 78, 90, 110, 116, 119, 120, 122, 126, 132, 138, 214

Photo © Steve Pool pages 25, 39, 96, 98, 100, 102, 103, 104, 106, 108, 140, 147, 150, 152, 154, 155, 156, 159, 163, 165, 167, 169, 171, 175, 179, 183, 184, 189, 191, 192, 194, 199, 200, 201, 203, 206, 207, 208, 211

Photo © Raphael Buchler pages x, 136

All other photos licensed by Shutterstock

About the Author

An award-winning journalist with experience in many markets as a local television anchor and reporter, Dari Alexander is currently the main anchor for Fox 5 News in New York City, with an average of three million viewers each night. A reporter for Fox News for ten years, she has also anchored *Fox & Friends* and *Fox News Live* hours. Alexander also trained as a chef in New York and Paris, where she learned how to create recipes that are both delicious and healthy. She lives in New York City with her husband and two children.

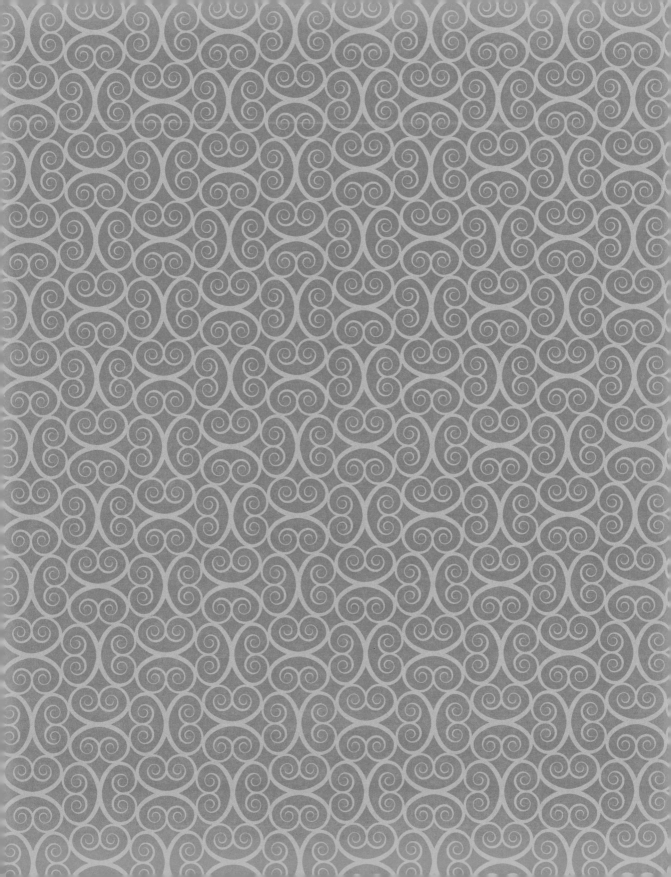